The Veterinary Care of the Horse

The Veterinary Care of the Horse

Sue Devereux and Liz Morrison

J. A. Allen
London

British Library Cataloguing in Publication Data

The veterinary care of the horse
I. Title   II. Morrison, Liz
636.1089

ISBN 0–85131–543–7

First published in Great Britain in 1992 by
J. A. Allen & Company Limited
1 Lower Grosvenor Place
London SW1W 0EL

Reprinted 1993
Reprinted 1994
Reprinted 1995
Reprinted 1996
Reprinted 1998

Designer: Nancy Lawrence
Production editor: Bill Ireson
Typesetting: Waveney Typesetters, Norwich, Norfolk
Printed and bound in Great Britain by The Bath Press, Bath

Contents

Acknowledgements

The authors of this book would like to thank the numerous people who assisted with its production. Our special thanks go to Rebecca Hamilton-Fletcher, BVSc, MRCVS, and Sarah Stoneham, BVSc, MRCVS, who gave advice and encouragement at every stage.

We are also indebted to several members of the Bristol University Veterinary School and Lt-Col John Hickman, MA, FRCVS, for their help and advice, and to June Morrison for preparing the index.

We would like to thank:

T. R. C. Greet, BVMS, MVM, FRCVS, for use of the photographs in Figures 14.8 and 14.9.

M. H. Hillyer, BVSc, MRCVS, for use of the photographs in Figures 12.2 and 12.4.

J. G. Lane, BVetMed, FRCVS for the use of the photograph in Figure 14.10.

F. G. R. Taylor, BVSc, PhD, MRCVS, for use of the photographs in Figures 10.3, 10.4, 12.5, 12.6 and 14.7.

A. I. Wright, BVSc, MRCVS, for use of the photographs in Figures 15.4, 15.5, 15.6, 15.11, 15.12, 15.13 and 15.26.

The British Veterinary Association for permission to reproduce the certificate used in Figure 19.1.

We thank all of the following friends and clients who allowed us to photograph their horses or assisted in providing the subjects for photography:

Mr B. Bladon, BVMS, MRCVS
Brympton Riding School
Catherston stud
Miss L. Clarke
Mrs P. Crozier-Cole
Mr R. S. Cull, BVetMed, MRCVS
Mrs S. M. Cutts
Mrs G. Davies
Mrs C. A. East-Rigby
Grovely Riding School
Miss M. Gurdon
Hurdcott Livery Stables
Mrs P. Jamieson
Mrs S. Kenworthy
Miss B. Miller
Lady J. Norman-Walker
Mr J. D. Puzio, BVetMed, MRCVS
Ms A. Schardt
Skers Farm
Ms J. Smith
Mrs A. Standen
Mrs S. Tate
Mrs C. Thomas
Mr D. Townsend
Miss S. Venton
Miss S. Warwick
Miss T. Weal
Mrs G. Wheeler
Whitcombe Manor Racing Stables
Mr J. Woodhall, BVetMed, MRCVS
Mrs E. Woolley
Mrs T. Yarrow

Finally, we would like to thank Graham Devereux and Graham Wilson for their help and moral support throughout the time it took to complete the book.

Introduction

Everyone who owns or looks after horses builds up a basic knowledge of injuries and medical conditions. This includes knowing when to call the vet out, how to cope in an emergency and the way to nurse a sick or injured horse back to health.

The Veterinary Care of the Horse has been written to add to this knowledge. The aim is to help owners, riders and grooms understand the vet's approach and provide the best of care for their horses.

The text is written in a style which makes information on any subject easy to find. The book covers the common conditions that vets are called upon to treat. Clear guidance is given on the immediate course of action required and when to seek professional help.

It is important to remember that the symptoms of any condition can vary from horse to horse. Therefore, the vet in attendance will make the diagnosis and determine the most suitable treatment which may differ from that outlined in the text.

1 Preventive Medicine

The Healthy Horse

It is important to be familiar with the signs of good health, so that any illness can be detected in the early stages.

The signs include:
- attitude – bright, alert, with pricked ears and taking an interest in the surroundings
- appetite – good
- coat – shiny with healthy skin
- eyes – bright with no discharge
- nostrils – clean
- condition – good without being fat
- droppings – passed regularly and break on hitting the ground. Depending on the diet, the normal colour is greenish-brown or golden brown
- temperature – between 37 and 38 °C (98.5 to 100.5 °F)
- pulse – 30 to 40 beats per minute
- respiration rate – 8 to 16 per minute. The horse's breathing should be barely noticeable.

Memorising these signs will help you to recognise when a horse is ill. If you have any doubts about the horse's health, you should always consult your vet.

Preventive medicine

Preventive medicine comprises the routine procedures that are carried out to keep the horse in good health and to protect it from disease.

These procedures include:
- vaccination against tetanus and equine influenza
- a worming programme
- teeth rasping
- shoeing and hoof care
- prompt attention to any injuries or changes in the horse's health.

Planning ahead

Missing any of these important procedures can prevent the horse from working and prove to be an expensive oversight. It is therefore advisable to plan the worming programme and book visits for vaccination, dentistry and shoeing in advance. Mark the appropriate dates in a diary or calendar.

Do not forget retired horses and brood mares, as they require the same consideration and veterinary care. They are equally at risk even though they rarely leave the field.

Minimising the cost

Whether you keep the horse at home or in a yard, it is more cost effective to arrange for a shared visit. Some veterinary practices offer a discount for routine treatment of large groups of horses.

Vaccination

Vaccines are available to protect horses and donkeys against equine influenza and tetanus. Owners should ensure that all the animals in their care are vaccinated.

Vaccination programme

The recommended vaccination programme which complies with both the Jockey Club and FEI rules is as follows:

Primary course

Two injections of a combined influenza and tetanus vaccine with an interval of 4–6 weeks.
   N.B. Maximum immunity is not achieved until two weeks after the second injection.

6 month booster

An influenza booster is required six months after the second injection of the primary course.

12 month booster

An influenza and tetanus booster is given six months later, i.e. 12 months after the second injection of the primary course.

Programme options

Once the recommended programme is complete, influenza boosters must be given at intervals of no longer than 12 months. Tetanus boosters are needed every 18–30 months.
   One of the following schedules should be adopted:

12 monthly boosters

Basic course – total of four injections, then
Booster 1 – influenza
Booster 2 – influenza and tetanus
Booster 3 – influenza
Booster 4 – influenza and tetanus

9 monthly boosters

Basic course – total of four injections, then
Booster 1 – influenza
Booster 2 – influenza
Booster 3 – influenza and tetanus
Then repeat the sequence.

6 monthly boosters

If outbreaks of influenza occur, or the horse is at high risk of exposure to infection (e.g. competition horses), the frequency of vaccination can be increased to intervals of six months, e.g.
Basic course of four injections, then
Booster 1 – influenza
Booster 2 – influenza
Booster 3 – influenza
Booster 4 – influenza and tetanus
The sequence is then repeated.

Remember only healthy horses should be vaccinated. If a horse is coughing or off colour, inform the vet *before* the vaccine is given.

Exercise following vaccination

Wherever possible, vaccinations should be given at the start of a rest period. This is because although the majority of horses appear to suffer no ill effects from the vaccine, some are definitely below par for a few days. Occasionally a horse becomes quite ill.

For a horse that is in work the following guidelines are suggested:

- do not travel or tire the horse immediately prior to vaccination
- following each of the two *primary* vaccinations, the horse should not travel or be worked hard enough to make it sweat for seven days. Ridden walking exercise and turning out can be continued as normal
- following *booster* injections the horse should not be worked hard or travel for 3–4 days
- when side effects occur, notify your vet and do not work the horse at all.

Pregnant mares

Pregnant mares should be given an influenza and tetanus booster 3–6 weeks prior to foaling to give the foal maximum protection. Antibodies are passed to the foal in the colostrum; this is known as 'passive immunity'.

Foal immunisation

Foals should begin their primary vaccination course when three months old. Until this age they are still protected by the maternal antibodies.

There is no point in vaccinating the foal before the passive immunity wanes, as the antibodies prevent the vaccine stimulating an immune response.

Orphan foals and those born to unvaccinated mares should be given tetanus antitoxin within two days of birth. This is different from the vaccine; it gives immediate, short-acting protection.

A second injection 3–4 weeks later helps protect them until the full programme is started at three months of age. If the foal is injured, the injection should be repeated.

The Jockey Club ruling

All horses entering racecourse premises, whether for a show, Pony Club camp or a sponsored ride, must be vaccinated in accordance with the Jockey Club rules.

These state that:

1) All horses and ponies must receive a primary course of two vaccinations against equine influenza. These are given 21–92 days apart.
2) The first booster must be given 150–215 days after the second injection of the primary course.
3) Subsequent booster injections should be at intervals of not more than one year.
4) When starting a new vaccination course, the horse is allowed to compete and enter competition premises from seven days after the second vaccination. The horse does not have to wait for the third injection at 150–215 days.
5) No horse is allowed to compete or enter competition premises until seven days after any influenza vaccination.

The rules are different for horses born before January 1, 1980, in that:

- they are not required to have had the third dose of vaccine 150–215 days after the second dose
- the booster interval before March 16, 1981 must not exceed 14 months.

FEI Rules

The FEI ruling differs only in that the booster between 150 and 215 days is not compulsory.

Vaccination certificates

Vaccination certificates now include a diagram and written description of the horse which must be completed by a veterinary surgeon. This is to ensure that the documented injections have been received by the horse described.

Make sure the certificate is kept up to date. If a booster is overlooked and is given more than 12 months after the last injection, the horse will have to begin the programme again.

Many show organisers insist that these certificates are shown before allowing entry to the ground. This rule reduces the chance of an infected animal entering the ground and spreading the virus.

When purchasing a new horse, always ask for the vaccination certificate. If it is not available or not up to date, start a new programme.

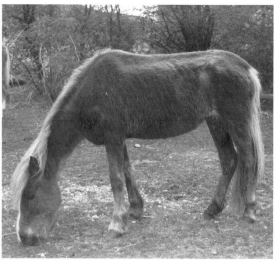

Figure 1.1 *This pony shows the weight loss and ill-thriftiness often associated with a high worm burden*

Worm Control

In large numbers, worms can cause a variety of clinical signs, ranging from loss of condition (*Figure 1.1*) to death of the horse. Worms are one of the most common causes of colic.

It is, therefore, necessary to adhere to a strict programme of worming and pasture management.

Clinical signs

Some of the common equine worms and the symptoms they cause are listed in *Figure 1.2*.

The horse may be infected by more than one type of worm. The damage is caused by the feeding habits of the adult worms and the migratory activity of the larvae. This is illustrated by examining the life cycle of the large redworm, *Strongylus vulgaris* (*Figure 1.4*).

Diagnosis

Diagnosis is made on:
- the clinical signs
- the grazing and worming history
- examination of the faeces for worm eggs.

A negative worm egg count does not always exclude worms as the cause of the problem. For example, if the horse has recently been wormed, very few adult worms remain to produce eggs. The horse may still be infected by large numbers of larvae unless a larvicidal drug was used.
- blood tests – anaemia and a raised eosinophil count are suggestive of worm infestation. When migrating *Strongylus vulgaris* larvae are causing damage, the beta$_1$ globulin is raised
- post mortem examination of the gut.

	Large Redworm Strongylus vulgaris	Small Redworm Trichonema spp.	Roundworm Parascaris equorum	Tapeworm Anoplocephala perfoliata	Threadworm Strongyloides westeri	Pinworm Oxyuris equi	Lungworm Dictyocaulus arnfieldi	Bots Gastrophilus spp.
Adult Size (cm)	1.4–2.4	0.4–2.6	15–50	up to 8	up to 0.9	0.9–1.5	3.6–6	1.8
Location of Adult Worm in Host	Caecum Colon	Caecum Colon	Small intestine	Ileum Caecum	Small intestine	Caecum Colon Rectum	Bronchi of lungs	Free-living insect
Location of Larvae in Host	Intestinal arteries	Caecum Colon	Liver Lungs	Forage mite is intermediate host	Lungs and other tissues	Caecum Colon	Lymph vessels Lungs	Stomach Pharynx
Host Age Group Affected	All ages	All ages	Mostly under 3 yrs	All ages	Foals	All ages	All ages	All ages
Range of Clinical Signs	anaemia anorexia weight loss poor performance reduction of growth rate rough coat diarrhoea colic death	anaemia anorexia weight loss diarrhoea colic death	anorexia ill-thrift pot belly emaciation diarrhoea colic bowel obstruction coughing nasal discharge	often no clinical signs in large numbers may cause intussusception and death	weight loss ill-thrift diarrhoea	intense anal irritation tail rubbing	chronic cough especially during exercise nasal discharge increased respiratory rate	gastric ulceration

Figure 1.2   *Clinical signs caused by common equine worms*

Treatment and prevention

Worms can be controlled by a combination of regular worming, with careful choice and administration of treatments, and good pasture management.

The worming programme

Frequency of dosing

In spring and early summer, horses should be wormed every month. This is because the eggs hatch quickly and larvae migrate rapidly from the droppings to the pasture.

From late summer onwards, the interval between treatments can be extended to six weeks. It should not exceed six weeks or there will be a sharp rise in egg output (*Figure 1.3*), resulting in pasture contamination.

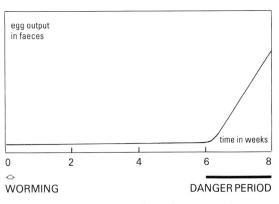

Figure 1.3   *Diagram to show the increase in worm egg output when the worming interval exceeds 6 weeks*

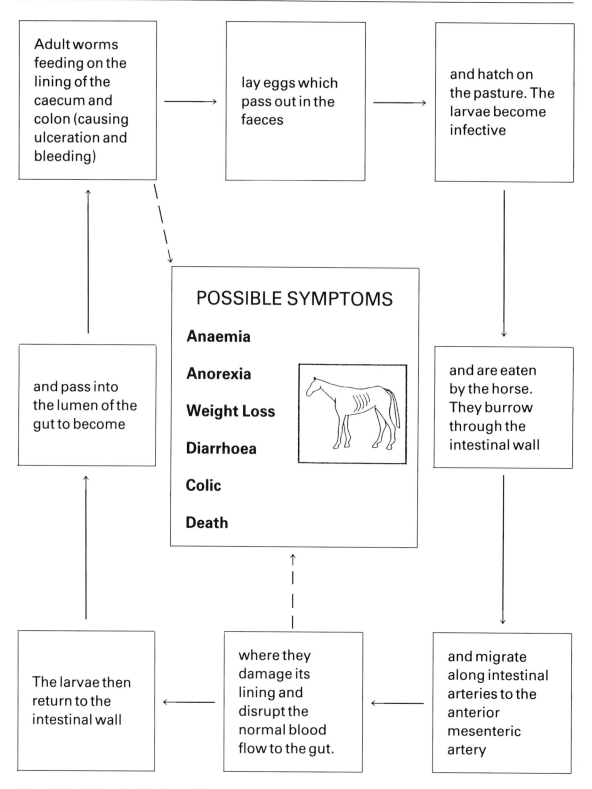

Figure 1.4   *Life cycle of the large redworm,* Strongylus vulgaris

Occasional dosing (i.e. 2–4 times a year) achieves very little. Although the majority of adult worms are killed and the number of worm eggs contaminating the pasture is temporarily reduced, the benefits are short-lived:
- within 6 weeks, more larvae have developed into adults and the egg output rises again
- the horse is continually being reinfected by larvae already on the pasture.

If *every horse in the field* is treated at 4–6 week intervals, the larval population on a contaminated field will gradually decline. Over a 12 month period it reaches acceptable levels.

Potential hazards

The success of a worming programme can be spoiled by a variety of factors, but two of the most important are missed treatments and resistance of the worms to certain drugs.

Missed treatments

A single horse that misses a treatment puts all the others at risk. A horse with a worm egg count of 1,000 e.p.g (eggs per gram of faeces) releases 15 million eggs a day onto the pasture.

Resistance

Many strains of small redworm are known to have become resistant to some drugs in the benzimidazole group. This means that the adults are not killed and the egg output continues, despite regular administration of these worming preparations.

These problems will be detected if the droppings of each horse are tested at regular intervals.

Choice of worming preparation

Worming preparations (*Figure 1.5*) are called *anthelmintics*. There is a wide choice on the market.

No drug kills every type of worm. The choice of drug therefore depends on whether it is being used to treat a specific problem or as part of a routine control programme.

Change of anthelmintic

Whenever a new anthelmintic is used, the droppings should be tested two weeks later.

If the worm egg count is negative, the preparation can be used for one year.

If the worm egg count is positive, the worms may be resistant or the horse may have been underdosed. Discuss the situation with the vet who will advise you of the appropriate action to take.

The following year, use a drug from a different chemical group. *Avoid changing the drug too often as this can encourage resistance.*

If the chosen preparation is not effective against bots, give a single dose of a suitable wormer in November.

Administration of treatment

Working out the dose

Horses are dosed according to their bodyweight (*Figure 1.6*). (Instructions are always printed on the packet.) The vet will help you estimate the horse's weight.

Drug safety

It is important to remember that underdosing does not kill the worms and may encourage resistance.

Ivermectin, pyrantel embonate and the

Drug	Brand name	Large Redworm Adults	Large Redworm Larvae	Small Redworm	Roundworm	Tapeworm	Threadworm	Pinworm	Lungworm	Bots	Stomach Worm
Ivermectin	(Eqvalan)	++	++	++	++	−	++	++	++	++	++
Pyrantel Embonate	(Strongid P)	++	−	++	++	++ Double dose	−	++	−	−	−
Organophosphorus Compounds Haloxon	(Multiwurma)	++	−	++	++	−	−	++	−	++	−
Benzimidazole Drugs Fenbendazole	(Panacur)	++	++* *8 × dose or normal dose for 5 days	++R 4 × dose	++	−	++ 7 × dose	++	++ Double dose	−	−
Mebendazole	(Telmin)	++	−	++R	++	−	−	++	++ Double dose for 5 days	−	+
Thiabendazole	(Equizole)	++	−	++R	++ Double dose	−	++	++	−	−	−
Oxibendazole	(Equitac) (Equidin)	++	−	++	++	−	++ 1.5 × dose	++	−	−	−
Oxfendazole	(Systamex) (Synanthic)	++	++	++R	++	−	−	++	−	−	++

Figure 1.5 *Efficacy of different anthelmintics:*
++ = *effective.* − = *no activity or not tested*
R = *resistant strains reported*

benzimidazoles are all very safe drugs. Horses will tolerate several times the recommended dose without experiencing any harmful side effects. If in doubt, err on the generous side when estimating a horse's weight.

Organophosphorus drugs are the exception and the recommended dose should *never* be exceeded. They are also unsuitable for certain groups of horses, so check the data sheet before use.

Always rest the horse the day after worming. When large numbers of adult worms or larvae are killed, the impact on the gut is likely to make the horse feel off colour.

Paste or Granules?

Some manufacturers offer a choice of either a paste which is administered by syringe directly into the mouth, or granules which are mixed in the feed. Both are equally effective.

Type of animal	Height in hands	Weight in kg
Shetland pony	9–10	140–180
Donkey	9.2–11	150–250
Child's pony	12	300
Arab	14–15	380–450
Thoroughbred	15–17	450–600
Hunter	15.2–17.2	500–650
Heavy hunter	16+	700
Shire	17+	up to 1,000

Figure 1.6 *Approximate bodyweights of adult horses, ponies and donkeys*

To administer a *paste*:
1) Adjust the syringe to give the required dose.
2) Put a headcollar on the horse and make sure there is no food in its mouth.
3) Push the nozzle gently in through the side of the horse's mouth and towards the back of its tongue.
4) Depress the plunger and remove the syringe.
5) Hold the horse's head up to prevent it spitting out the dose.
6) Check that none of the dose has been wasted.

- Advantages: paste is usually quick to administer.
- Disadvantages: a few horses object to the treatment. If any of the dose is wasted, the amount must be estimated and an additional dose administered.

To administer *granules* mix them into the feed. Molasses or carrots can be added to increase palatability.
- Advantages: granules are often slightly cheaper than paste.
- Disadvantages: feeding must be supervised to ensure the whole dose is consumed. If the horse rejects the feed, the treatment is wasted.

Worming of foals

Foals are particularly susceptible to worms. They should be dosed monthly from four weeks of age.

Ideally, foals should only graze fields which have not been used by horses for at least a year.

Pregnant mares

Pregnant and lactating mares must be wormed every 4–6 weeks.

Most preparations are safe but the instructions on the packet should be checked carefully before administering *any drug* to a pregnant mare.

Pasture management

The best methods of reducing pasture contamination are:
- ploughing and reseeding
- resting it from horses for at least a year.

If this is not possible, the grazing can be improved by other means:

Anthelmintic strategy

- Every horse in the field must be wormed at the same time.
- The interval between dosing should not exceed 4–6 weeks.
- New horses must be treated and have a negative worm egg count before going into the field. (If the droppings are not tested, wait three days before turning the horse out to allow the eggs to clear.)
- All horses should be wormed before moving onto fresh pasture.
- Routine egg counts should be done each spring and whenever the anthelmintic is changed.

Removal of droppings

Removal of droppings twice a week is a very effective method of reducing the number of larvae on the pasture.

Horse paddocks can be divided into close-cropped grazing areas and patches of long, sour grass where the horses pass their droppings. The larval contamination of the rough areas is much higher than the rest of the field.

If the droppings are removed before the

eggs hatch and the larvae migrate onto the pasture, the contamination is significantly reduced. The grazing area can be increased by up to 50 per cent.

Harrowing

Harrowing should be done during a warm, dry spell of weather so the faeces and larvae dry out quickly.

When done in warm damp conditions, it simply spreads the infective larvae into the grazing area.

Mixed grazing

Grazing horses with cattle and sheep is generally overrated as a method of worm control.

The stomach worm, *Trichostrongylus axei*, is common to sheep, cattle and horses. Without a suitable worming programme, cross infection can occur.

Teeth Rasping

Being a herbivore, the horse spends most of its day chewing the hard, vegetable material which makes up its food. It chews with a circular action of the lower jaw, relying on its teeth to break up the food into small particles suitable for swallowing.

To compensate for the constant wear, the permanent teeth of the horse (*Figure 1.7*) grow throughout its life.

Reasons for teeth rasping

The cheek teeth in the upper jaw of the horse are set wider apart than those of the lower jaw. As a result, sharp ridges or spikes develop on the inside edge of the lower teeth and the outside edge of the upper teeth (*Figure 1.8*). These spikes can be razor-sharp. If they are not removed, ulcers may develop on the inside of the horse's cheeks and on the edges of its tongue.

A horse's teeth should therefore be rasped by a vet or equine dentist at least once a year.

Signs that the teeth need rasping

These include:
- loss of condition
- quidding – partially chewed food is dropped from the mouth
- eating slower than usual
- resentment of the bit or schooling problems.

Inspecting the teeth

Horses should have their teeth inspected every six months because some will need their teeth rasped more than once a year.

This procedure should always be done with *extreme care*. Do not attempt it when the horse has food in its mouth.

Upper cheek teeth

1) Stand in front of the horse and gently but firmly grasp the tongue through the interdental space on one side of the mouth.
2) Slide the forefinger or index finger of your free hand inside the cheek on the opposite side and feel the outer edge of the upper premolars.
3) Be as quick and as gentle as possible and take care not to be bitten. Repeat the procedure, checking the other side of the mouth.

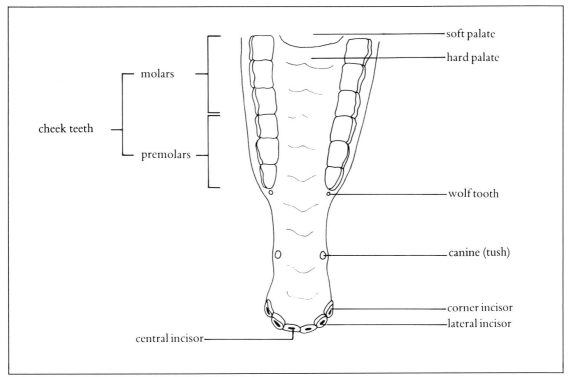

Figure 1.7   *The permanent teeth in the upper jaw*

Lower cheek teeth

1) Never attempt to feel the inner edges of the lower teeth.
2) Visual inspection using a torch or when facing the light will reveal any sharp edges.

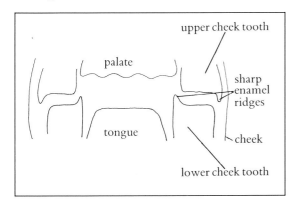

Figure 1.8   *Vertical section through a horse's mouth showing the wear of the cheek teeth*

Even if the premolar edges are smooth, do not allow more than twelve months to elapse between each rasping as the posterior molars may have sharp edges.

Preparing for tooth rasping

Before the vet arrives, make the following preparations:
- do not feed the horse or its teeth will be covered with food material
- have the horse ready in a stable, wearing a headcollar with a loose noseband. If the headcollar is too tight, it prevents the horse's mouth being opened fully. It also causes the rasp to bruise the horse's cheeks as it passes underneath the tight straps
- the vet will require an assistant, a bucket of clean water, a towel and a brush for cleaning the rasps.

The procedure for teeth rasping

The vet will inspect the horse's mouth and then instruct you how to hold the horse. The teeth are then rasped to remove all the sharp edges. Some horses resent the procedure and require a twitch or sedative.

Removal of 'caps'

The premolar milk teeth are replaced by permanent premolars when the horse is between two and a half and four years of age.

A milk tooth is sometimes retained and sits like a cap on top of the permanent tooth. This should be removed by the vet before it causes the tongue or cheeks to become sore.

Wolf teeth

Small teeth with short roots may be found in the upper jaw, in front of the first premolar. These are known as wolf teeth. They have no function and are not present in every horse.

Problems caused by wolf teeth

In many cases, the wolf teeth cause no problem at all and should be left alone.

However, they can be knocked by the bit, resulting in inflammation of the gum. They may also be very sharp or angled in such a way that they ulcerate the cheeks.

Extraction and aftercare

Wolf teeth are usually simple to remove and should be extracted if there is any suspicion that they are causing a problem.

Following extraction, the horse should not be ridden for up to a week while the gum heals and any bruising subsides.

2 The Injured Horse

First Aid

The management of the injured horse is broadly divisible into two key areas: immediate first aid and the ongoing treatment of injuries.

The first-aid kit

Every yard should have a first-aid kit (*Figure 2.1*) which contains the materials likely to be needed to treat an injury.

It should be kept in a clean tin or covered plastic box, in a relatively dust free area such as a cupboard. Items must be replaced as they are used. The kit should contain:

Clean bowl
Clean towel
Large roll of cotton wool
Curved scissors
Bactericidal skin cleanser, e.g. Hibiscrub or Pevidine
Ready-to-use poultice, e.g. Animalintex
Antibacterial cleansing cream, e.g. Dermisol
Non-stick dressing, e.g. Melolin
Gauze
Lint
Pack of sterile saline solution
Large syringe
A selection of bandages and tape, e.g. 2 stretch gauze bandages (7.5 cm/10 cm)

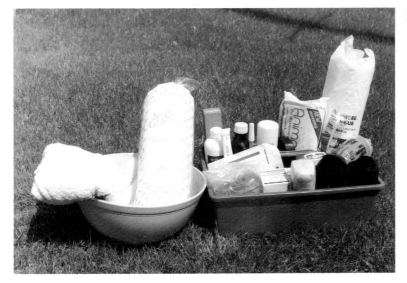

Figure 2.1   *The first-aid kit*

2 conforming elastic bandages
1 crepe bandage
Adhesive or self-adhesive bandage, e.g.
Elastoplast or Vetrap
Tubular bandage, e.g. Tubigrip
1 set of stable bandages
1 roll electrical insulating tape
1 roll parcel tape
Roll of padding, e.g. Gamgee
Wound powder
Antibacterial and anti-inflammatory oint-
ment, e.g. Dermobion
Gentian violet and antibiotic spray
Petroleum jelly, e.g. Vaseline
Tube of antibiotic eye ointment
Small pair of tweezers or forceps
Thermometer
Paper and pencil
Tourniquet, e.g. an old tie.

Managing a Wound

The healing of a wound is influenced by the
way it is managed *immediately* after an accident occurs.

Whether you decide to call the vet or to
treat the injury yourself, a systematic approach should be adopted.

Immediate action

1) Control the bleeding.
2) Assess the injury and call the vet if necessary.
3) Protect the wound from contamination
and further injury.
4) Assess the degree of shock.
5) Clean the wound.
6) Control infection.
7) Prevent or reduce swelling.

The importance of the above procedures
cannot be over-emphasised and it is worth
looking at each of them in more detail.

1)　To control bleeding

Any wound which is bleeding profusely
looks very alarming, but *do not panic*.

First, assess the flow of blood:
- a cut vein results in a steady, gentle flow of
blood.
- a cut artery emits a jet of blood in time with
each heartbeat.

Significant blood loss occurs only when
haemorrhage from a large artery or vein is
left uncontrolled.

Although stopping the bleeding is the first
priority, *try not to contaminate the wound further*. If at all possible, wash your hands and
use clean materials.

The methods used to control bleeding all
rely on applying *pressure*.
- bandage a non-stick dressing (e.g. Melolin) and a pad of clean Gamgee over the
wound
- if the site cannot be bandaged, place the
pad over the wound and hold it firmly in
place. The bleeding usually stops after a
few minutes. If it does not, reapply the
pressure
- bleeding from a single damaged artery can
be stopped by pressing the skin firmly
about an inch above the vessel. This can be
done while the first-aid kit is fetched
- with leg injuries, a tourniquet may be used
to control severe arterial bleeding while
waiting for the vet. It is placed above the
wound with a pencil or smooth stick
underneath it. The pencil is then twisted to
tighten the tourniquet until the bleeding
stops
- while the tourniquet is in place, put a
pressure bandage over the wound. The
tourniquet *must* be loosened every 10 minutes to allow blood to flow through the
lower limb. It should be removed as soon
as the bleeding is under control.

2) Assessing the injury

Many small cuts and grazes can be cleaned and treated without calling the vet.

Always call the vet if:
- the wound is large or deep
- the bleeding cannot be controlled
- the wound is very dirty
- the horse is in pain
- considerable swelling develops
- you suspect a foreign body
- the horse shows signs of shock
- tetanus injections are not up to date
- you are uncertain how to proceed.

Keep the horse warm.

Apply essential first aid.

Clean (hose) the wound if it is dirty.

Where applicable, arrange transport for the horse.

Boil water and leave it to cool in a clean container.

Have some means of restraint available, e.g. a bridle.

Carry out any instructions given by the vet over the phone.

Figure 2.2   *Seven things to do while waiting for the vet*

3) Protecting the wound

Once bleeding is under control, take steps to minimise further contamination or damage. Straw, wood shavings, dust, mud and flies all introduce *infection*, which delays healing.

If the horse has to be walked through mud or transported in a vehicle which contains bedding, bandage a non-stick dressing and a pad of Gamgee over wounds below the knee or hock.

Stand the horse on a clean, hard surface while preparing to treat the wound.

Do not apply topical medication (e.g. wound powder or ointment) at this stage, especially if the wound is likely to be sutured (stitched). Some preparations are irritant and actually delay healing.

4) Managing a shocked horse

Following an accident, a horse may show signs of shock. These include:
- trembling
- fast and shallow breathing
- cold clammy skin
- a low temperature
- faint pulse due to low blood pressure.

Always call the vet as shock usually indicates a serious injury or severe pain.

5) Cleaning the wound

Thorough cleaning of any wound is essential. It should be done in an area with good light and a clean floor so wood shavings or straw do not enter the wound.

If the wound is very painful, the horse may need to be restrained. The vet may give a sedative.

Before the vet arrives, hose off any mud, straw, etc. If the injury is on a limb, begin hosing below the wound. Gradually work upwards while quietly reassuring the horse. Make sure that dirty water from around the wound does not run onto the damaged tissue.

Continue hosing until the wound is clean, then protect it with a clean dressing and a firm support bandage to minimise the swelling.

Cleaning procedure

If you have decided to treat the wound yourself:
a) Wash your hands.
b) Use curved scissors to trim away any hair overhanging the wound edges, taking care not to let it fall into the wound.
c) Clean the skin around the wound with warm water and a bactericidal soap, e.g. Hibiscrub. Use cotton wool or gauze swabs. Dirty water should not be allowed to run onto the injured tissue.
d) Clean the wound with boiled water that

has cooled or sterile saline. Begin at the centre of the wound and work outwards. Discard each swab as soon as it is dirty – never put it back into the clean bowl of washing solution. Forceps or tweezers may be used to remove foreign material.

e) Finally, rinse the clean wound with sterile saline solution, using a syringe.

Strong antiseptics should not be used as they can damage the exposed tissues. With minor wounds such as scratches and grazes, a very dilute solution of Hibiscrub, Savlon or Pevidine may be used.

Once the wound has been cleaned, reassess the injury. Where necessary, the cleaning procedure can be continued by application of either:
- a poultice, e.g. Animalintex
- a cleansing cream, e.g. Dermisol.

You may decide to call the vet at this stage if dirt is embedded in the wound or it is more extensive than originally supposed. The vet will trim away any damaged tissue and give further treatment.

6) The control of infection

The risk of infection is reduced by:
- immediate treatment
- thorough cleaning
- maintaining cleanliness
- use of antibiotics, either topically (applied directly onto the wound) or systemically (a course of treatment is given orally or by injection).

Antibiotics can only be prescribed by a vet.

7) The control of swelling and pain

Excessive soft tissue swelling should be prevented where possible as it:

- impedes the circulation of blood through damaged tissues
- makes the tissues more difficult to suture
- puts strain on the suture line which can cause the wound to break down.

After cleaning and treatment, the swelling can be prevented or reduced by:
- bandaging
- light exercise in hand
- administration of non-steroidal anti-inflammatory drugs, e.g. phenylbutazone. This drug is also a powerful analgesic. Reducing the pain encourages the horse to use the injured leg.

Your vet will make recommendations taking into consideration the site and nature of the wound and the individual horse's reaction to the injury.

Wound Healing

Any damage to living tissue – whether a cut, a bruise or a sprain, results in *inflammation*.

Inflammation is a vital part of the repair process. The blood supply is increased and white blood cells migrate from the blood into the tissue. They ingest dead tissue, bacteria and foreign material.

The period of exudation lasts for up to five days. During this time, most wounds undergo a degree of contraction and the skin edges are drawn closer together.

Over the next 7–10 days, the inflammatory exudate is replaced by proliferating *granulation tissue*. This consists of collagen fibres and capillaries. The dividing epithelial cells at the skin edges migrate across this bed of healthy tissue to close the wound.

The growth of new skin is a very slow process. It proceeds at an approximate rate of

0.5 to 2 mm a day. For this reason, wounds are sutured wherever possible.

Suturing

Suturing a wound leads to rapid healing with the smallest possible scar. Closing the skin edges minimises the amount of new tissue required to heal the defect. This is known as *first intention healing*. The tight covering of skin stops the development of proud flesh.

Even if skin has been lost and the wound can only be partially sutured, the healing time is greatly reduced.

Wounds cannot be sutured if:
- there is extensive skin loss
- the wound is contaminated by grit, hair, etc.
- bacterial infection is present
- the blood supply to a flap of skin has been lost.

Suturing is therefore done at the discretion of the vet, following close inspection of the wound.

If all is well, the sutures are removed after approximately 10 days. However, sutured wounds sometimes break down. This is usually due to foreign material or infection in the wound. The skin edges are no longer in apposition and healing proceeds by granulation. This is *second intention healing*.

Healing of open wounds

Problems often arise with wounds that cannot be sutured or have broken down.

Wounds on the head and trunk are difficult to bandage and must be kept very clean. Clean paper is the most suitable bedding.

Open wounds below the knee and hock heal very slowly due to:
- poor blood supply
- low temperature

- minimal wound contraction as the skin is tightly bound to the underlying tissues
- susceptibility to contamination and infection
- swelling
- proud flesh.

These problems can be minimised by appropriate use of bandages and dressings.

Wound dressings

Excessive use of creams, powders and ointments can impair healing.

During the early stages of open wound healing, the following dressing materials are recommended:
- gauze squares impregnated with petroleum jelly or antibiotic, e.g. Jelonet or Fucidin Intertulle
- Gamgee or cotton wool
- a conforming type of bandage.

The gauze does not stick to the wound. Exudate passes through the dressing and is absorbed by the Gamgee. The bandage keeps the dressing in place and provides compression which controls swelling and proud flesh.

N.B. Petroleum jelly impregnated dressings should only be used for the first 3–4 days as prolonged use may encourage the development of proud flesh. Change to a dry dressing, e.g. Melolin.

Managing proud flesh

When granulation tissue grows above the level of the skin, it is called proud flesh (*Figure 2.3*). The tissue is usually lumpy, pink and shiny. It may have a yellowish tinge and it bleeds very easily.

The tissue can mushroom out of the wound. This acts as a physical barrier, preventing skin growth and closure of the wound.

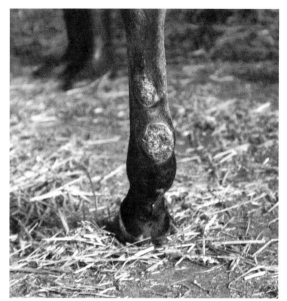

Figure 2.3   *Proud flesh*

sulphate crystals. These may be used alone or mixed with an antibiotic powder or cream. Vaseline should be used to protect the surrounding skin. The copper sulphate is bandaged in place for up to 12 hours. When used with care it is very effective.

3) Surgical removal

This is carried out by the vet. Local anaesthesia is not required as there are no nerve endings in granulation tissue. The proud flesh is trimmed to below the skin level using a scalpel. The tissue bleeds freely and the haemorrhage is controlled by a pressure bandage.

4) Skin grafting

Where there is a large area of skin loss or a recurrent problem with excessive amounts of granulation tissue, a skin graft may be required.

Small pieces of skin are removed from the horse's neck, flank or thigh. They are embedded in the healthy granulation tissue at 1 cm intervals. The majority of the grafts will fail, but each surviving piece of skin produces a hormone called the 'epithelial growth factor'. This stimulates the division of epithelial cells and inhibits development of proud flesh.

There are several methods of managing proud flesh, so veterinary advice is essential.

1) Application of a corticosteroid cream

The cream or ointment may also contain an antibiotic. It is applied once or twice a day under a non-stick dressing and a firm bandage.

In most cases, treatment is effective. However, corticosteroids can also inhibit the growth of epithelial cells at the skin edges and its long term use can prevent the wound from healing.

2) Application of caustic substances, e.g. copper sulphate

Copper sulphate destroys proud flesh, but it also damages the delicate epithelial cells at the wound margin. The proud flesh is covered with a thin layer of finely ground copper

5) Leaving the wound uncovered

Opinion varies on whether wounds benefit from being left completely open and exposed to the air. With sites such as the *head and trunk* which are difficult to bandage, there may be no choice.

All *lower limb* wounds need to be covered until the defect has filled in with healthy granulation tissue.

Where healing is proceeding satisfactorily, it is advisable to leave the dressings on. Where proud flesh keeps developing, the vet may suggest leaving the wound uncovered for part of the day.

The proud flesh is trimmed and the wound is kept bandaged only until the bleeding has stopped. Initially, the trimming may need to be repeated every couple of days.

The wound must be kept as clean as possible.

When the horse remains stabled:
- move it to a box with no bedding for most of the day
- skip out every couple of hours
- feed soaked hay from a net to reduce the dust. Regularly remove uneaten hay from the floor
- cover the wound with a light dressing, e.g. Tubigrip, before returning the horse to its usual stable.

Do not turn the horse out with the wound unprotected:
- in dusty or muddy fields
- in the fly season.

The important thing to remember is that no two wounds are the same and they change from day to day. If you are concerned by lack of progress, or if the prescribed treatment is no longer working, contact your vet.

Treating minor cuts and grazes

Simple cuts and grazes usually heal well if left open, provided they are not contaminated by mud or bedding.

The following steps should be taken:
- clean the wound thoroughly
- apply an antibacterial powder, spray or cream
- examine the wound twice daily
- check for secondary bacterial infection which can develop unnoticed beneath a crust of wound dressing and exudate. If pus is present, remove the scab and clean the wound before applying more dressing.

Dressings

The type of dressing is a matter of personal preference or availability. In the summer, a dressing with an insect repellant is recommended.

Wound powder

This is puffed onto the wound from a small plastic container. It is easy to apply and adheres well to a moist surface.

Do not use near the horse's eyes. When treating a head injury, puff the powder onto a piece of cotton wool before applying it to the wound.

Aerosols and sprays

These are convenient to use and are useful for scratches and small grazes.

If the horse dislikes the noise, spray the preparation onto cotton wool first. Never spray near the eyes.

Creams and ointments

These do not stick to moist wound surfaces. Dust and other pieces of debris can adhere to them.

Puncture wounds

Puncture wounds are made when small, sharp objects, e.g. nails, thorns, etc., pierce the skin.

The object may penetrate to quite a depth and deposit bacteria and foreign material deep in the tissues.

Cleaning the wound properly is difficult because the wound is deep with a small skin opening. There is a tendency for the hole to heal over, leaving dirt trapped in the tissue. This can lead to infection and abscess formation.

Treatment

It is advisable to call the vet as the risk of infection is high and antibiotic treatment is often required.

The following steps need to be taken:
- remove any visible foreign body
- apply a poultice if practicable
- where poulticing is not possible, foment the wound for 15 minutes, two or three times daily
- keep the wound open
- check that the horse's tetanus vaccinations are up-to-date.

Haematomas

A haematoma is a blood blister that develops under the skin.

It can develop following:
- a kick or a blow
- intramuscular injections given into the brisket. The needle sometimes damages a blood vessel as it passes through the skin and superficial layers of muscle.

Blood leaks from the damaged vessel and accumulates under the skin forming a swelling which is usually soft and painless. It may be very large. The swelling tends to move downwards slowly over the next few days.

Treatment

Treatment is not usually necessary. Most haematomas diminish in size and disappear within 1–2 weeks.

Large or persistent haematomas should be seen by the vet.

Poulticing

Hot poultices are applied to:
- dirty wounds
- infected wounds
- puncture wounds
- developing abscesses.

They act in two ways:
- the warmth increases the blood supply to the injured area. The white blood cells help clear away bacteria and other debris
- fluid is drawn from the wound. Small foreign bodies may also be drawn out.

Potential problems

There are two dangers to avoid:
- the poultice must not be so hot that it burns the tissue. Test the temperature of the poultice with the back of your hand before applying it
- the securing bandage *must not be too tight*. Its purpose is simply to hold the poultice in place. Remember that wet bandages can shrink and tighten as they dry.

Types of poultice

All poultice materials are covered with a layer of polythene after application. This helps to retain the heat and ensures that fluid is drawn from the wound rather than from the atmosphere.

Poultices should be replaced every 12 hours.

The most common types of poultice include:

Animalintex

This consists of a thick layer of padding, impregnated with bassorin and boric acid. One side of the padding has a polythene backing.

The dressing is cut to size and placed in a shallow tray. It is saturated with clean, hot water and then squeezed as dry as possible. The poultice is applied to the wound with the polythene facing outwards. It is held in place with cotton wool or Gamgee padding and a bandage.

Kaolin

This is supplied in a tin. The lid is loosened and the tin is heated in a pan of hot water until the contents are hand hot. The kaolin is then spread onto a piece of Gamgee, covered with several layers of gauze and applied to the injured area. It is retained with a bandage.

Magnesium sulphate paste

This is used in the same way as kaolin. It is available in 500g tubs or small 50g pots suitable for one or two dressings.

Kaolin and magnesium sulphate paste are particularly suitable for foot injuries. They should not be applied directly onto an open wound.

Bran and Epsom salts

This poultice is also used for foot injuries. A handful of Epsom salts is added to a scoop of bran. Sufficient boiling water is added to make a crumbly (not wet) mixture, and the poultice is applied when cooled to the correct temperature (hand hot).

Steps in poulticing the foot

1) Prepare all the materials you will need.
2) Stand the horse on a clean surface.
3) Clean and dry the *whole foot* thoroughly.
4) Apply the poultice and waterproof covering.
5) Secure it with a bandage or suitable boot, e.g. an Equiboot.
6) Keep the horse in, on a thick, clean bed.

Packing the foot

When the poultice is in place, pack the concavity of the sole with pads of Gamgee. The outer couple of pads should extend beyond the sole to cover the weight-bearing edge of the hoof wall. These pads may be kept in place with an old sock.

The packing has three functions:
- it keeps the poultice firmly in contact with the wound, ensuring maximum efficiency
- the pressure on the sole forces pus out of the hole when the foot bears weight
- the padding beneath the hoof wall reduces the wear on the covering bandage, especially if the horse is shod.

Securing the dressing

Secure the dressings with Elastoplast or Vetrap. Completely cover the sole and wall of the hoof. When using Vetrap or bandaging over a sock, include the heels and coronary band to stop the dressing slipping off. Elastoplast used alone sticks securely to the hoof wall and and should not be in contact with the coronary band.

For extra strength, wrap a layer of the

covering bandage around the lower edge of the hoof wall so half the width can be turned in under the sole. Repeat this a couple of times.

Wide parcel or carpet tape can also be used to reinforce the dressing and make it waterproof.

Using an Equiboot

An Equiboot (*Figure 2.4*) is useful for holding sole dressings in place. The concavity of the sole is packed with Gamgee and the top layer

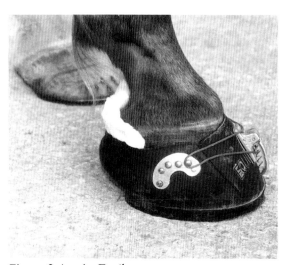

Figure 2.4   *An Equiboot*

is cut long enough to cover the bulbs of the heels.

Equiboots are available in six sizes. They are adjustable and are sold with fitting instructions. A badly fitting boot can cause painful rub injuries.

Hot fomentation

This is a method of applying heat to an area that cannot be poulticed. It should be done for 20 minutes, two or three times a day.
- half fill a bucket with hand-hot water
- add a double handful of Epsom Salts
- immerse a small towel in the water
- squeeze out the excess, fold the towel in four and apply to the wound or abscess
- after a couple of minutes, repeat the procedure
- top up the bucket with boiling water to keep it hot.

Hot tubbing

This is useful for punctures and bruises of the sole.
- pick out the hoof and scrub it clean
- add a handful of Epsom salts to a half-filled bucket of warm water; the temperature should be comfortable for your hand
- place the hoof in the bucket and keep it immersed for 10–15 minutes
- add more hot water as the temperature cools
- repeat the procedure twice daily
- dry the leg thoroughly afterwards.

Bandaging

Bandaging is a skill which is acquired with practice. Selection of appropriate dressings and bandages keeps the wound clean and dry but still allows adequate ventilation.

Bandages provide:
- warmth
- support
- compression (which inhibits proud flesh)
- protection from:
  – bacterial infection
  – contamination

– desiccation (drying out)
– further injury

A correctly applied bandage gives light, even pressure. It is firm enough to hold the dressings in place but does not restrict the circulation.

Overtight bandages can cause pressure sores, skin sloughs (*Figure 2.5*) or tendon damage.

Loose bandages are ineffective and can be dangerous.

Important points to remember

- Bandages should always be applied over a layer of padding, e.g. Gamgee or cotton wool. This helps to distribute the pressure evenly.
- Any lumps or creases in the padding must be smoothed out.
- Overlapping half the width of the bandage each time ensures even pressure.
- The ties or velcro fastenings on elastic bandages should be laid flat and be *no tighter* than the bandage. Knots must be tied at the *side* of the limb to avoid pressing on the tendons at the front and back of the leg.
- For extra security, the ends may be covered with electrical insulating tape or Elastoplast. This should completely encircle the leg and stick back on itself.
- If the horse bears less weight than normal on the injured limb, put a support bandage (*Figure 2.6*) on the opposite leg.

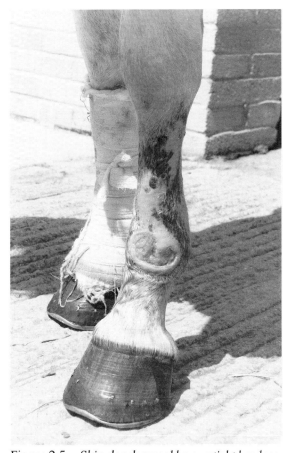

Figure 2.5 *Skin slough caused by overtight bandage*

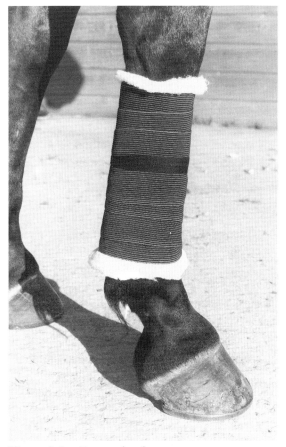

Figure 2.6 *Support bandage*

Applying a support bandage

To put a support bandage on the lower limb of a horse (*Figure 2.7*), follow these steps:
1) Cover the wound with a non-stick dressing.
2) Use a stretch gauze bandage to hold the dressing in place. Begin on the side of the limb and wrap the bandage around the leg before spiralling down over the dressing and back up to the starting point. The pressure should be light and even.
3) Wrap Gamgee or cotton wool twice around the leg. The padding must extend from just below the knee or hock to the fetlock.
4) Use a conforming elastic bandage, Vetrap or Elastoplast as the support bandage. Unwind it in the same direction as the overlap of the padding. Start halfway down the cannon bone, placing the end of the bandage under the flap of the padding. Spiral once around the limb, work down to the fetlock, then back up to just below the knee or hock and finally down to the starting point. The pressure should be firm enough to provide support *without restricting the blood supply*.
5) Check the bandage regularly to ensure it is comfortable and secure.

If the pastern is to be included, in addition to the above points:
• use the stretch gauze bandage to secure additional padding at the back of the pastern
• wrap the double layer of padding around the limb so that it extends from the knee or hock to the coronet
• proceed as before with the outer bandage, but continue over the fetlock joint to include the pastern.

Signs that the bandage is too tight

The signs to look for which will indicate that

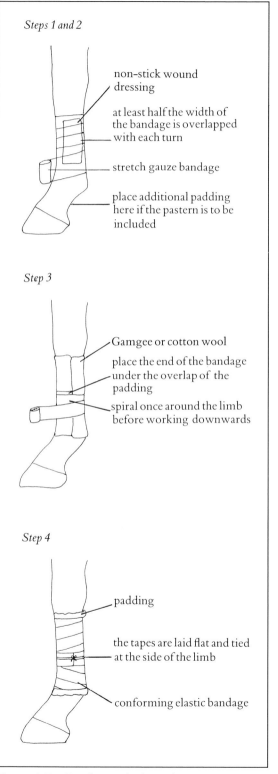

Steps 1 and 2

non-stick wound dressing

at least half the width of the bandage is overlapped with each turn

stretch gauze bandage

place additional padding here if the pastern is to be included

Step 3

Gamgee or cotton wool

place the end of the bandage under the overlap of the padding

spiral once around the limb before working downwards

Step 4

padding

the tapes are laid flat and tied at the side of the limb

conforming elastic bandage

Figure 2.7   *Bandaging the lower limb*

the bandange is too tight include:
- swelling above or below the bandage
- signs of discomfort from the horse (e.g. lifting the leg or biting the dressing)
- areas of skin that are sore to touch when the bandage is removed.

Using a pressure bandage

A pressure bandage is used for short periods of time to control bleeding. It is applied in the same way as a support bandage but with firmer pressure. It should be loosened after 15 minutes except under veterinary instruction.

Bandaging a small coronet wound

Electrical insulating tape, 20–25 mm wide, is ideal for bandaging a small coronet wound (*Figure 2.8*). Follow these steps:
1) Cut a non-stick dressing and a piece of Gamgee to a size that just covers the wound.
2) Stick the end of the insulating tape on the hoof wall just below the coronet and wrap it around the hoof to secure the lower edge of the dressing.
3) Pass the tape around the hoof again but bring it up over the dressing and then back onto the hoof wall.
4) Continue until the dressing is completely covered. Avoid sticking the tape directly onto the coronary band.

N.B. The hoof wall must be clean and dry.

Bandaging a heel wound

1) Cut a non-stick dressing and a piece of Gamgee to cover the wound.
2) Attach the free end of a roll of insulating tape to the hoof wall. Wind the tape round the hoof, passing below the heels to secure the lower edge of the dressing.
3) Pass the tape round the hoof wall again. This time bring it up over the dressing on the heel and then back down onto the hoof wall.
4) Repeat two or three times until the dressing is secure.
5) Avoid direct contact between the tape and the coronary band.
6) Wind a short length of crepe bandage twice around the bulbs of the heels and the coronary band.
7) Secure the crepe bandage with two or three layers of Elastoplast (*Figure 2.9*).

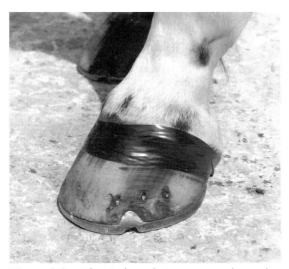

Figure 2.8 *Electrical insulating tape can be used to bandage a small coronet wound*

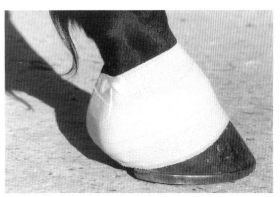

Figure 2.9 *Bandaged heel wound. Electrical insulating tape may be used on top of the Elastoplast for additional security*

Bandaging the foot

See earlier in this chapter, Poulticing.

Bandaging the knee and hock

These are awkward sites to bandage as the constant movement tends to loosen the bandages. They can then slip down the leg and cause undesirable ridges of pressure.

Tubular bandage

These problems can be eliminated by using a tubular bandage (*Figures 2.10 and 2.11*). This bandage is slipped over the foot and secured above the knee or hock with Elastoplast.

It holds the dressing in place and does not need to be removed each time the dressing is

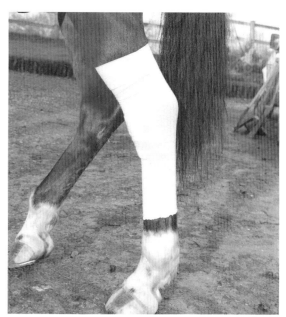

Figure 2.11   *Hock dressing held in place by a tubular bandage*

changed. The lower edge of the bandage is simply rolled up to allow cleaning and inspection of the wound.

Zip fastening bandages

Zip-up elastic support bandages (e.g. Pressage) are available for the knee and hock joints. If one of the standard sizes fits your horse, they can also be used to keep dressings in place.

Conventional bandaging techniques

The knee

Wound dressings applied to the knee may be held in place by use of a 7.5 cm stretch gauze bandage in a figure-of-eight pattern (*Figures 2.12 and 2.13*).

Follow these steps:
1) Place a non-stick dressing and a double layer of Gamgee over the wound.

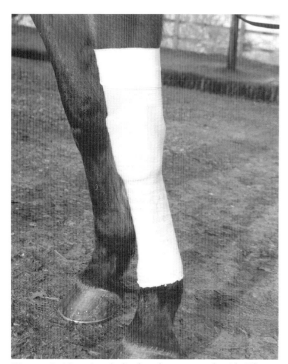

Figure 2.10   *A tubular bandage secured with Elastoplast can be used to hold knee dressings in place*

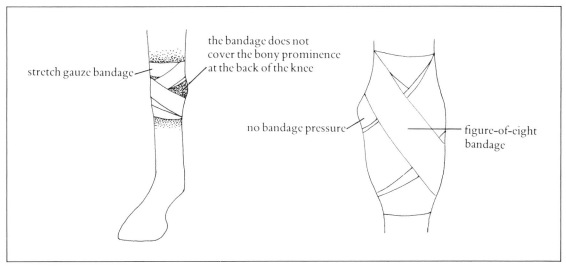

Figure 2.12 *Bandaging the knee:* (left) *side view;* (right) *front view*

2) Wind the bandage two or three times around the leg so that the lower edge of the bandage is just above the bony prominence at the back of the knee. This secures the upper border of the dressing.
3) Proceed with a figure-of-eight bandage. Avoid covering the bony prominences behind the knee and on the inside of the upper knee. Keep the pressure light and even.

Check with your vet whether further padding is required and the best method of securing it. If the injury is such that the bony prominences must be covered, additional padding is used with holes cut over the pressure points.

Elastoplast can be used to prevent the bandage slipping. It is applied over the bandage and adheres to the skin above and below the knee. Take care, as repeated application can make the skin sore.

Finally, apply a support bandage to both front legs.

The hock

It is very difficult to bandage the hock with-

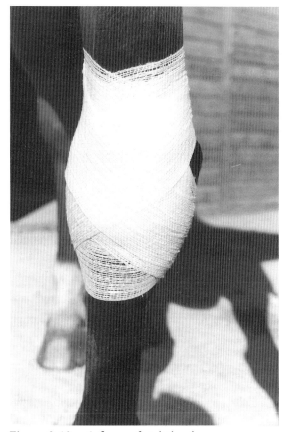

Figure 2.13 *A figure-of-eight bandage*

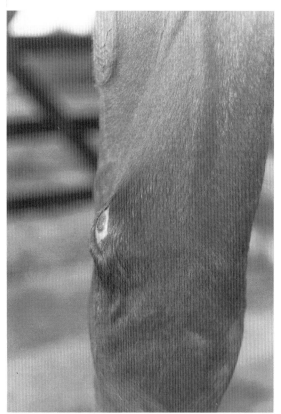

Figure 2.14   *Pressure injury from an incorrectly-applied bandage*

out putting unwanted pressure on the Achilles tendon, the point of the hock or the bony prominence on the inside of the joint.

If a hock injury needs bandaging, you should seek veterinary advice.

How to stop a horse removing bandages

This problem can be overcome in a number of ways:

Comfort

Check the bandage to ensure that it is not too tight and causing discomfort. Reapply it if necessary.

Application of unpleasant tasting substances

Smear the substance, e.g. Cribbox, liberally over the surface of the outer bandage. This method is messy but it usually works. Some horses learn to accept the bandage after a few days.

Wearing a bib

A bib (*Figure 2.15*) is a bowl-shaped device

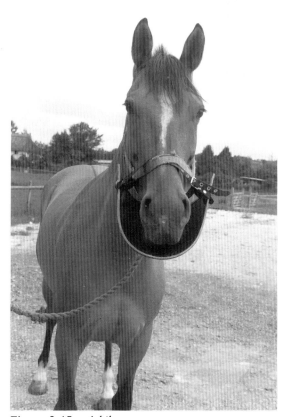

Figure 2.15   *A bib*

made of strong plastic that is strapped to the headcollar noseband and prevents the horse nibbling the bandages. The horse is still able to drink and pull hay from a net.

Wearing a cradle

A cradle (*Figure 2.16*) consists of several rounded rods of wood, joined together with strong plastic string. The device is strapped

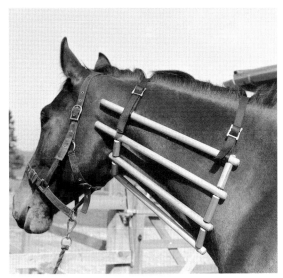

Figure 2.16   *A cradle*

around the horse's neck. It allows some movement but restricts flexion. The horse is unable to bend its neck and remove the bandages.

Wearing a muzzle

A muzzle (*Figure 2.17*) effectively stops a horse removing its bandages but will also

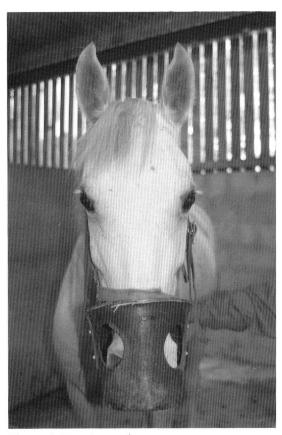

Figure 2.17   *A muzzle*

prevent it eating. Make sure the horse has learnt how to drink with the muzzle in place before leaving it on for any length of time.

3 Examination of the Lame Horse

The Lame Horse

There are many causes of lameness and this chapter outlines the procedures that may be used in order to make a diagnosis. The seven chapters that follow cover most of the problems commonly encountered.

Some of the conditions described do not always cause immediate lameness. In many cases, prompt veterinary attention can prevent the problem becoming more serious.

It is the owner's or groom's responsibility to be familiar with the normal appearance and feel of the horse's limbs and to seek specialist advice if any change is noticed.

Definition of lameness

The 'normal' conformation and action of horses varies considerably. Lameness can be defined as any change from the horse's usual way of moving. It is therefore necessary to be familiar with each individual horse's action.

Whether slight or severe, lameness is usually a sign of pain. The horse must not be worked until the problem has been investigated and the cause identified.

When to call the vet

The following guidelines are suggested to help you decide when to call the vet. *Immediate* attention must be given to horses which are:
- unable to bear any weight on a limb
- unable to move
- trembling and sweating due to pain.

Also those that have:
- very swollen limb(s)
- puncture wounds of the foot
- obvious wounds

In other cases it is reasonable to wait a day or two to see if there is any improvement before seeking veterinary advice. In the meantime, it is essential to:
- rest the horse
- check very thoroughly for wounds and swellings on the legs
- search for nail or flint penetrations of the feet
- note any changes. If the lameness becomes worse or does not improve, call the vet.

Never ignore a slight lameness or swelling because the horse has an event in the near future. No occasion is worth the gamble of turning a minor problem into a more serious injury.

Preparation for the vet's visit

In advance of the vet's arrival:
- bring the horse in
- make sure the stable is clean
- have a headcollar or bridle ready

- pick out the hooves and clean the legs
- think carefully about the history of the case and write it down.

Steps of the examination

The cause of the problem is sometimes obvious to both the owner and the vet, but on other occasions a considerable amount of diagnostic work is required to pinpoint the site of pain. The examination procedure varies with the individual situation. The vet will undertake some of the following steps:

Taking the history

It is helpful to the vet if you consider the answers to the following questions in advance of the visit.

Timing

How long has the horse been lame?
Is this a recurrent problem?

Possible causes

Has the horse fallen or been kicked?
When was it last shod?
What was it doing when the problem was first noticed?

Exercise

What sort of exercise routine has been followed?
When is the lameness most marked?
Does the lameness improve or become worse with exercise?

Swellings

Have any swellings been observed?
If so, do they increase or decrease with exercise?

Stance

Is one foot pointed or rested more than the other?
Does the horse shift its weight from one foot to the other?

Examination at rest

Valuable information may be obtained by observing the horse at rest in the stable. The vet will look at the overall conformation and stance of the horse, and check for signs of pain. At the same time the history of the case will be discussed and questions asked as appropriate.

Trotting up

Unless the source of pain is obvious, the horse is walked and trotted up on a hard, flat surface. If it is necessary to use the road, the horse should always wear a bridle to ensure maximum control.

The handler should stay level with the horse's shoulder and allow complete freedom of the head. Placid or lazy animals should be driven on from behind, as pulling on the reins or holding them too short can prevent the slight head movements which aid identification of the lame limb.

Horses with forelimb lameness lift their heads up as the lame limb contacts the ground. The head drops as the sound limb takes the weight.

With hind limb lameness the horse is best viewed from behind. The hip on the affected side rises as weight is taken on the leg. The hip on the opposite side sinks as the sound limb bears weight.

Flexion test

A flexion test may be performed after the

trotting up. This involves picking up the horse's limb and holding it flexed for a period of 1–1.5 minutes. The horse is then asked to move straight into trot.

Increased lameness for the first few strides suggests the problem may lie in one of the flexed joints. The opposite limb is flexed for comparison.

N.B. Older horses often show stiffness or slight lameness for the first few strides following flexion.

Lungeing

Some types of lameness only become apparent when the horse is worked on a circle. In these cases, lungeing on hard and soft surfaces becomes a necessary part of the examination.

Examining the limbs

By this stage the vet will have identified the affected limb. This is closely examined and compared with the opposite leg. The vet will check for swelling, heat or pain and any muscle wasting will be noted.

Detailed examination of the foot

Where appropriate, the foot will be examined and compared with its opposite for:
- size and shape
- heat
- wear on the shoes
- obvious defects.

A thin layer of horn may be scraped from the sole to check for bruises and punctures.

Hoof testers are applied all round the sole and wall to test for any areas of particular sensitivity. If the vet suspects the presence of corns or bruising at the white line, the shoe will be removed.

Further tests

When the cause of lameness is not revealed by the examination, further tests are necessary to establish and confirm a diagnosis. These are normally carried out at a later appointment.

The procedures the vet may use include:
- nerve blocks
- radiography (x-rays)
- ultrasound scanning
- faradic assessment.

(For details of these techniques see Chapter 19.)

4 Conditions of the Foot

Anatomy

By far the majority of lameness is the result of foot injury or disease. Some knowledge of the horse's anatomy is necessary for an understanding of the various problems that can arise.

Throughout this section, the authors have purposely used the anatomical terms that are in everyday use within equestrian circles. B.H.S. examination candidates and readers wishing to learn the modern nomenclature are referred to *Figure 4.1.*

The horse's foot consists of the protective hoof and all the structures it contains.

The hoof is modified skin. The wall, sole, frog and periople are derived from the epidermis; the underlying sensitive laminae and the sensitive tissues of the sole, frog, periople and coronet are derived from the dermis.

Name used in text	Alternative names
pedal bone	distal phalanx (third phalanx, coffin bone)
short pastern	middle phalanx (second phalanx)
long pastern	proximal phalanx (first phalanx)
coffin joint	distal interphalangeal joint
navicular bone	distal sesamoid bone
white line	white zone
pastern joint	proximal interphalangeal joint
fetlock joint	metacarpophalangeal joint – forelimb metatarsophalangeal joint – hind limb
cannon bone	third metacarpal bone – forelimb third metatarsal bone – hind limb
splint bone	second (medial) and fourth (lateral) metacarpal/metatarsal bone
knee	carpus
hock	tarsus
tibiotarsal joint	tarsocrural joint

Figure 4.1 *Anatomical nomenclature*

External Structures

The periople, the hoof wall, the sole, and the frog make up the external structures of the foot (*Figures 4.2 and 4.3*).

Periople

The periople is a band of soft, pale grey horn

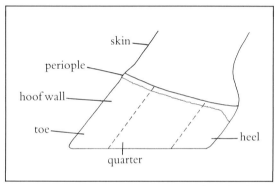

Figure 4.2   *The external structures of the hoof, side view*

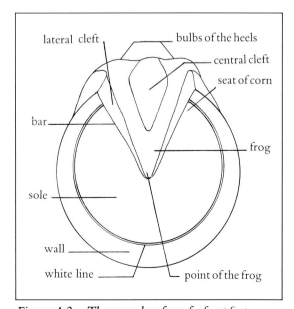

Figure 4.3   *The ground surface of a front foot*

which extends a variable distance down the hoof wall.

It bridges the junction between the skin and the hoof wall and is widest at the heels, where it merges with the frog.

It has the important function of restricting evaporation of moisture from the horn.

Hoof wall

The hoof wall extends from the coronary band to the bearing (ground) surface. It is divided into the *toe*, the *quarters* and the *heels*.

The wall is thickest at the toe, where most protection is needed, becoming thinner and more elastic towards the heels.

It is reflected forwards from the heels to form the *bars*, which can be seen when the foot is viewed from the ground surface.

The internal surface of the hoof wall has approximately 600 *horny laminae* which run vertically along its length. Each of these leaf-like structures has 100–200 secondary laminae. These interdigitate with the *sensitive laminae* which are attached to the periosteum of the *pedal bone*. This interlinking of the sensitive and insensitive laminae holds the pedal bone firmly in position.

Hoof growth

The hoof wall grows from the *coronary band* at the rate of 6–10 mm a month. It takes approximately six months for the horn at the coronet to reach the heels and 9–12 months to reach the toe.

Hoof rings

The wall is normally smooth, but variations of growth rate due to disease and dietary changes can cause horizontal rings to develop on the surface (*Figure 4.4*).

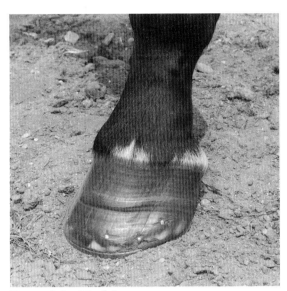

Figure 4.4 *Hoof ring*

The sole

The function of the sole is to protect the sensitive structures and to help support the weight of the horse. Its concave shape ensures that only the outer rim bears the horse's weight.

The thickness and concavity of the sole varies between individual horses. Some have thin, flat soles and are more prone to puncture wounds and bruising than those with thick, concave soles.

The area of sole between the wall and the bars is known as the *seat of corn*. This region is very susceptible to bruising.

The junction between the sole and the wall is called the *white line*. This narrow ring of soft, non-pigmented horn is a useful landmark for the farrier. It shows the thickness of the wall and indicates the position of the sensitive tissues which lie immediately inside it.

The frog

The frog is a triangular pad of soft, elastic horn which is normally in contact with the ground and plays an important role in reducing concussion. It has a central cleft and deeper clefts on either side.

The frog and sole are composed of horn which is softer than that of the wall and constantly flakes away.

Internal Structures

The internal structures of the foot (*Figure 4.5*) include the
- pedal bone
- navicular bone
- distal end of the short pastern bone
- coffin joint
- navicular bursa
- cartilages of the foot
- insertions of the:
  - deep digital flexor tendon
  - common digital extensor tendon
- digital cushion
- sensitive laminae
- ligaments, blood vessels and nerves.

The *coffin joint* lies between the pedal bone, the *short pastern* and the *navicular bone*.

The *deep digital flexor tendon* passes over the navicular bone and attaches to the pedal bone. Between the tendon and the bone lies the *navicular bursa*, a fluid-filled sac which cushions the movement of the tendon over the bone. The *common digital extensor tendon* attaches to the extensor process on the front of the pedal bone.

The *cartilages* of the foot (*Figure 4.30*) are attached to each side of the pedal bone. They project above the coronet and are easily palpated. They are normally springy, but as the horse ages, they can become hard and unyielding due to deposition of bone (*sidebone*).

The *digital cushion*, consisting of fibrous

and elastic tissue, occupies the space above the frog, between the two cartilages.

is transmitted to these supporting structures through the strong union of the sensitive laminae on the surface of the pedal bone and the insensitive laminae on the inside of the hoof wall (*Figure 4.5*).

The Function of the Foot

The horse's foot has three key functions:
- supporting the weight of the horse
- reducing concussion
- preventing slipping.

Supporting the weight

Most of the horse's weight is taken by the wall, the bars and the outer rim of the sole. It

Reducing concussion

Expansion of the frog and digital cushion plays an important role in absorbing concussion.

As the horse puts its foot to the ground, the weight is taken first by the frog and the posterior hoof wall. The frog expands and pressure is exerted through the digital cushion onto the flexible cartilages. These transmit the pressure to the relatively thin, elastic hoof wall at the heels, which in turn expands.

When there is no weight on the foot, the frog and digital cushion contract, allowing the foot to resume its resting conformation.

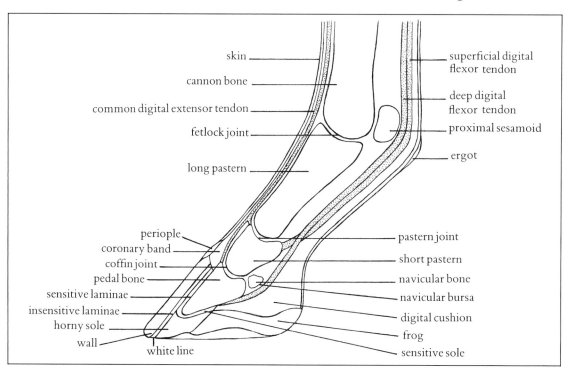

Figure 4.5   *Section through the lower limb and foot of the horse*

Preventing slipping

The triangular shape of the frog and the concave sole ensure that the feet are able to secure a firm hold on most types of going. The frog digs into soft ground, whereas the rim of the sole provides grip on hard, flat surfaces.

Routine Care

As the horse's foot is the commonest site of lameness, regular care helps to prevent problems.

Trimming

Trimming is required every 4–6 weeks. The farrier uses his skill to maintain or restore the correct hoof conformation. Without regular trimming, the hoof becomes split and misshapen.

Hoof conformation

When assessing hoof conformation and balance, the farrier will note the shape of the foot, and the thickness and quality of horn.

Side view

The hoof wall at the toe should be parallel to the hoof wall at the heel (*Figure 4.6(a), (b) and (c)*). The angle between the hoof wall and the ground should be 45–50 degrees in the forelimb (*Figure 4.6(a)*) and 50–55 degrees in the hind limb.

Excessively sloping conformation (*Figure 4.6(b)*) puts extra strain on the suspensory ligament, the sesamoids and the flexor tendons.

Very upright conformation (*Figure 4.6(c)*) leads to increased concussion and may predispose to the development of ringbone and arthritis of the lower limb joints.

Pastern/hoof axis

The pastern axis is an imaginary straight line joining the centre of the fetlock and pastern joints. It is continuous with the hoof axis which runs parallel to the anterior hoof wall between the coronary band and the ground.

The pastern/hoof axis should form an unbroken straight line, whatever the horse's conformation (*Figure 4.6(a), (b), (c) and (d)*).

If the pastern/hoof axis is broken (*Figure 4.6(e) and (f)*), i.e. the slope of the pastern and the anterior hoof wall are not the same, it should be restored to a straight line by corrective trimming of the hoof over a period of time.

Where the pastern/hoof axis is straight, but the hoof is more upright or sloping than normal (*Figure 4.6(b) and (c)*) it should not be altered by trimming the hoof.

Front view

In a horse with normal conformation, the toes point to the front. The pastern/hoof axis passes in a straight line through the centre of the fetlock and pastern joints and the centre of the toe (*Figure 4.6(g)*).

If the toes are turned in or turned out (*Figure 4.6(h) and (i)*), one side of the foot and lower limb is subjected to abnormal wear and strain. Special attention must therefore be paid to balancing the foot at each trimming or the problems will be compounded.

Where the pastern/hoof axis is broken as a direct result of hoof imbalance (*Figure 4.6(j)*

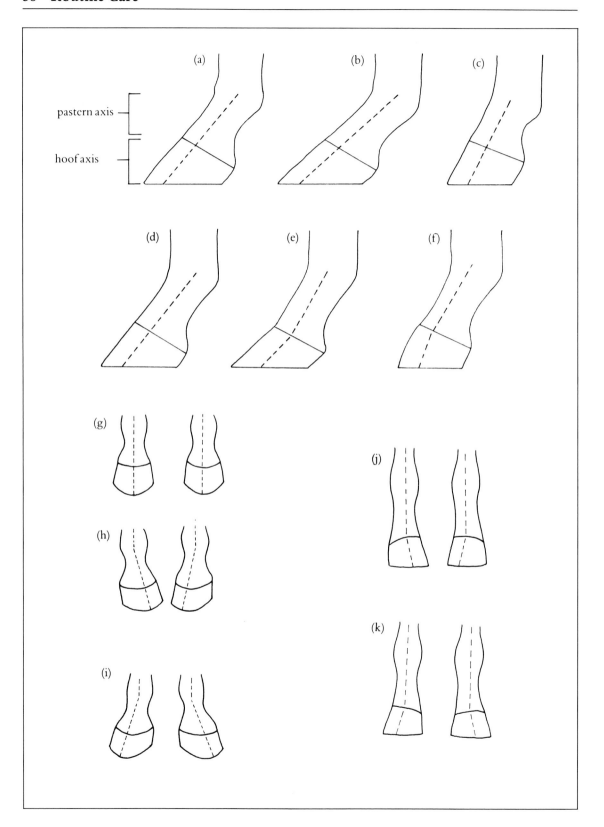

Figure 4.6 (opposite page) *Side and front views of the feet to show the pastern and hoof axes*

Side view:
Examples of: (a) normal; (b) sloping; (c) upright conformation with a straight pastern/hoof axis; (d) straight pastern/hoof axis; (e) and (f) broken pastern/ hoof axes. In (e) this can be corrected by trimming the toe and allowing the heels to grow. In (f) the heels should be lowered and the toe allowed to grow

Front view:
Examples of: (g) normal conformation; (h) toe-in conformation which puts abnormal strain on the outside of the limb and can predispose to lateral ringbone and sidebone; (i) toe-out conformation puts abnormal strain on the inside of the limb, predisposing to medial ring- bone and sidebone; (j) and (k) broken pastern/hoof axes due to foot imbalance. In (j) the medial wall is longer and should be trimmed. In (k) the lateral wall requires trimming

and (k)) it can be improved by appropriate trimming.

Ground surface

The medial and lateral hoof walls should be the same length. This can be checked by lifting the foot and viewing from directly above the heels. Imaginary lines drawn down the centre of the limb and across the heels should form 90 degree angles (*Figure 4.7*).

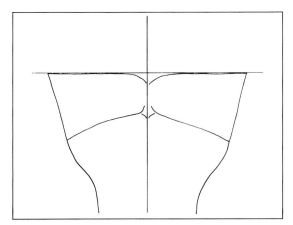

Figure 4.7 *Checking the hoof balance: the foot is lifted and viewed from directly above the heels*

Frog and heel conformation

The frog is not routinely trimmed as it should contact the ground and wear away naturally. However, loose flaps of horn which could trap debris in the clefts are removed.

Where the frog does not contact the ground, the heels tend to contract and the foot becomes smaller. This is undesirable and corrective action should be taken.

Sole conformation

In order to protect and support the sensitive tissues, the sole should be thick and concave.

Daily hoof care

- The feet should be picked out morning and evening and before and after exercise. Special attention should be paid to thorough cleaning of the clefts of the frog
- The shoe should be inspected for risen clenches and any movement away from the hoof wall
- The bedding of stabled horses must be kept clean and dry to prevent diseases such as thrush
- Ponies at grass in winter should have a well-drained area to stand on so the hoof does not become excessively soft and crumbly.

The value of daily applications of hoof oils and dressings is the subject of much discussion.

These oily preparations restrict the absorption and evaporation of moisture from the hoof.

They can be used to good effect on a fully stabled horse and during long spells of dry weather. Under these conditions the horn may become dry and brittle. Regular wetting of the feet restores the moisture balance of the horn and a coating of oil after the water has soaked in slows subsequent evaporation.

Shoeing

Shoeing protects the horse's feet from excessive wear. The shoes need replacing when the feet are trimmed every 4–6 weeks. After this time:

- the clenches begin to rise and can cause brushing injuries
- the shoe moves off the wall at the heels and may press on the seat of corn, causing lameness
- if a loose shoe is wrenched off, the nails can tear away large chunks of the hoof wall, making subsequent shoeing difficult
- the horse may tread on the nails of a cast shoe.

With some horses it can be false economy to remove the front shoes when they are turned away for a rest, especially during the summer months. The combination of hard ground and dry weather can result in cracking and excessive wear of the wall.

When horses are turned out without shoes the feet require trimming every 4 weeks.

Helping the farrier

Shoeing horses is very skilled and physically demanding work and a good relationship with the farrier should be developed. You can help in the following ways:

- book up the correct number of horses
- give advance warning if a particular horse is likely to be difficult and require extra time
- have the horses ready with clean legs and feet when the farrier arrives

- provide a swept, hard standing area with good light
- train your horses to let their feet be handled without leaning and fidgeting
- do not oil the feet before the farrier arrives.

Accidents associated with shoeing

Occasionally, a nail is driven too close to the white line (*Figure 4.8*). It may cause pressure on the sensitive laminae (nail bind) or penetrate the sensitive tissues (nail prick).

Nail bind and nail prick tend to occur when the wall is thin or the horse fidgets during shoeing.

Nail bind

Clinical signs

The horse usually becomes lame within a few hours of shoeing. However, symptoms may not develop for up to three days.

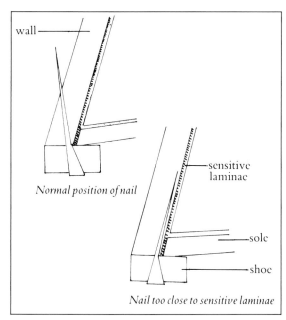

Figure 4.8 *Positioning the nail: (left) normal position; (right) nail too close to sensitive laminae*

Diagnosis

If the hoof wall is systematically tapped with a hammer, the horse will react when the offending nail is reached. The clench is often higher on the hoof wall than the others.

Treatment

- Ask the farrier or vet to withdraw the nail
- Rest the horse
- Poultice the foot for a couple of days.

Nail prick

Clinical signs

- The horse will jump and pull its foot away as the nail is accidentally driven into sensitive tissue
- There may be a little blood as the nail is withdrawn
- Lameness usually occurs immediately.

Treatment

This needs to be carried out as soon as the injury occurs.
- Flush the nail hole with an antiseptic solution such as iodine, or apply a poultice
- Bandage the foot and stable the horse
- Check that the horse is protected against tetanus
- If lameness persists, call the farrier or vet to open a drainage hole as an abscess may be developing
- Treat the foot as for a puncture wound.

Puncture Wounds and Pus in the Foot

Hoof punctures are a very common cause of lameness. Pus and gas result in a build up of pressure within the hoof, causing severe pain.

Causes

A flint or nail may penetrate the frog or sole causing bruising and haemorrhage of the sensitive structures. Bacteria and soil enter the hole and infection develops very quickly.

Clinical signs

These may include any or all of the following signs:
- slight lameness in the early stages, which progresses to:
  - minimal weight-bearing on the infected part of the foot, e.g. where there is an abscess near the heel, the horse takes most of its weight on the toe
  - refusal to bear any weight on the affected limb (*Figure 4.9*)
- increased heat in the foot
- an abnormally strong pulse in the digital vessels
- sweating, blowing and trembling if the pain is severe
- swelling of the flexor tendon sheath just above the fetlock. Less commonly, the swelling extends further up the limb
- a discharge of pus from the coronary band.

As pressure builds up inside the foot, the pus is forced along the path of least resistance. When there is no drainage hole, it runs under the sole and tracks up the white line. An area of the coronary band becomes swollen and tender before bursting to release the infection.

Diagnosis

Diagnosis is made following a thorough ex-

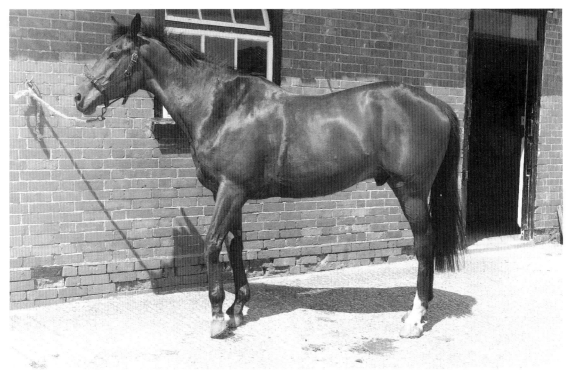

Figure 4.9 *A horse with pus in the foot is reluctant to bear weight on the affected limb*

amination of the foot. Where the site of penetration is not immediately obvious, the hoof is systematically squeezed with hoof testers to locate the tender spot.

Removal of the shoe is necessary when the white line is involved.

Immediate action must be taken if you suspect a horse has pus in the foot:
- call the vet or farrier
- clean the foot and look for any obvious wound
- check the horse's tetanus vaccination status
- apply a poultice and leave the horse stabled with a clean, dry bed.

Treatment

The aim of treatment is to drain the abscess and prevent reinfection.

Tetanus protection

If there is any doubt about the horse's vaccination status, tetanus antitoxin should be given. This is not a vaccine but it affords immediate protection for a short period of time while a full vaccination programme is initiated.

Drainage of the abscess

A portion of the sole is removed with a hoof knife to allow the escape of pus. This often brings immediate relief.

Elimination of infection

The *whole* foot should be thoroughly cleaned:

- scrub off any mud or bedding material
- tub the foot in a bucket of warm water with a handful of Epsom salts to draw out the infection
- flush the hole with a dilute solution of hydrogen peroxide to discourage the growth of anaerobic bacteria. Use an old syringe for this procedure
- wounds involving deep penetrations may require flushing with antibiotic solutions supplied by the vet
- poultice and bandage the foot. Protect it from moisture and dirt by using a water-proof covering or special boot.

Tubbing and poulticing is recommended once or twice daily until there is no more discharge. Occasionally the drainage hole closes prematurely and needs to be re-opened.

Antibiotics

Oral or injectable antibiotics are rarely necessary. They can *prolong* the period of lameness if administered when there is inadequate drainage.

They are likely to be prescribed:
- with deep penetrations of the foot
- where drainage has been established but the swelling of the leg increases or is slow to resolve
- to help prevent infection of fresh wounds that are detected and treated before any pus has formed.

Recovery

When there is no more discharge, the hoof should be covered with a dry dressing and inspected daily until new horn has grown over the sensitive tissues.

The sole may then be hardened by regular

applications of:
- a phenol, formalin and iodine mixture, or
- a gentian violet and antibiotic spray.

The horse should not be turned out until this stage has been reached.

Where the infection has been eliminated but the foot is still tender from bruising, a pad may be fitted under the shoe. This protects the newly healed sole from further injury. The pad is removed at the next shoeing.

Prognosis

The prognosis for uncomplicated abscesses and puncture wounds is good.

Deep Nail Penetrations

Deep nail penetrations of the foot are potentially serious, and the vet should always be consulted.

Special note

It is important to estimate the position and depth of the wound by observing:
- the length of nail inside the foot
- the angle of penetration.

Shallow penetrations in any area of the foot are unlikely to result in complications.

The risks associated with deep penetrations vary with the location of the nail. Consider a division of the foot into three areas (*Figures 4.10 and 4.11*).

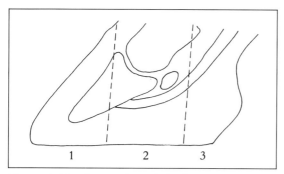

Figure 4.10   *Section through the foot*

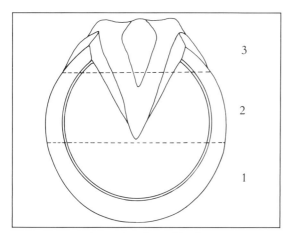

Figure 4.11   *Ground surface of the foot*

Penetrations in Area 1 may result in fracture or infection of the pedal bone.

Area 3 carries the least risk. The penetration would have to be very deep to damage the deep flexor tendon.

Area 2, the middle third of the foot, is the *danger zone*, especially when the frog or its clefts are penetrated.

Structures at risk include:
- the deep flexor tendon and its sheath
- the navicular bursa
- the navicular bone
- the coffin joint.

Frog injuries can be difficult to locate as the hole closes when the foreign body is removed. If you suspect a deep penetration of this region, call the vet at once.

Diagnosis

Diagnosis may involve specialised radiographic techniques. Contrast media (a fluid that shows up on x-rays) or a metal probe may be introduced into the hole enabling the extent of the penetration to be seen on x-rays (*Figure 4.12*).

Treatment

Treatment is likely to involve aggressive antibiotic therapy and surgery.

Prognosis

Penetration of the coffin joint or navicular bursa carries a very guarded prognosis. Fractures or infection of the pedal bone have a more favourable prognosis.

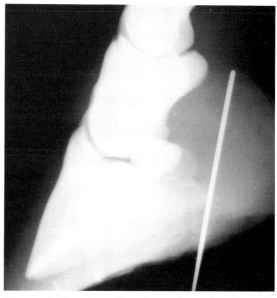

Figure 4.12   *A metal probe can be used to show the depth of a nail penetration of the foot on an x-ray*

Brittle Feet

In some horses the hoof wall and sole is comparatively thin and the rate of growth is abnormally slow. Despite regular trimming and shoeing, the walls tend to crack so securing a shoe becomes increasingly difficult (*Figure 4.13*).

The nails may have to be driven too close to cracks and previous nail holes, further weakening the wall.

Treatment/Prevention

The aim is to encourage the growth of good quality horn.

1) Feed a balanced diet

For example, use one of the complete diets with specified vitamin, mineral and protein levels.

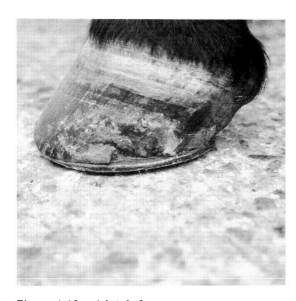

Figure 4.13   *A brittle foot*

The growth rate and quality of the horn may be further improved by supplementation with biotin, methionine or methyl-sulphonyl-methane (MSM). Multicomponent supplements are now available for horses with problem feet.

The supplement must be fed for at least five months before results can be expected. It is usually necessary to continue feeding the supplement for at least a year.

2) Have the feet regularly trimmed and shod

The shoes should be removed at the first sign of loosening to reduce the chance of being pulled off and further damaging the wall.

3) Ensure the horn does not become excessively dry

Approximately 25 per cent of the hoof wall is water. This needs to remain fairly constant for the horn to maintain its strength and elasticity.

Where the horn is too dry it becomes brittle and cracked; if it is too moist it becomes soft and crumbly.

A balance has to be established between evaporation and absorption of moisture from the hoof surface and the underlying sensitive tissues.

In dry weather, daily washing of the feet is beneficial. Use a sponge or soft brush so the protective periople is not scrubbed off. Apply oil to prevent evaporation once the water has soaked in.

4) Try to keep the horse in work

Exercise encourages horn growth. Avoid road work, hard ground and deep mud until sufficient good quality horn has grown for the shoe to be nailed on securely.

5) Stimulate the coronary band blood supply

Daily massaging with preparations such as Cornucrescine increases the blood supply and may improve the growth rate.

6) Prevent the entry of dirt and infection

Wide cracks or defects should be cleaned, dried and filled with an acrylic resin. As hoof repair materials can fall out at inconvenient times, ask your vet or farrier to demonstrate the technique. You will then be able to make temporary repairs to protect the hoof until their next visit.

7) Glue-on shoes

When the hoof wall is too weak for conventional shoeing, glue-on shoes (*Figure 4.14*) are useful.

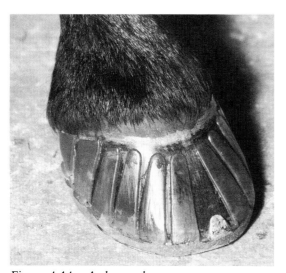

Figure 4.14   *A glue-on shoe*

The benefits are:
- the horse may be kept in work
- no nails are used, so the stress on the wall is reduced
- the hoof expands more naturally than with conventional shoes.

The disadvantages are:
- they are more expensive than ordinary shoes
- they are more time-consuming to fit
- they are more likely to come off if the horse is turned out.

Hoof Wall Cracks (Sandcracks and Grasscracks)

Hoof wall cracks that begin at the coronary band are known as *sandcracks*. Cracks that start at the ground surface and extend upwards are called *grasscracks*. They are described as toe, quarter or heel cracks according to their position.

These defects may be superficial, involving just the horn, or they may extend into the deeper, sensitive tissues. Heel and quarter cracks are more likely to cause lameness as the wall is thinner and the sensitive laminae are often affected.

Causes

There are a number of predisposing factors:
- failure to have the feet trimmed regularly. The hoof wall tends to spread and split as the feet lengthen (*Figure 4.15*)
- poor hoof conformation, e.g. long toes and low heels, or feet affected by chronic laminitis

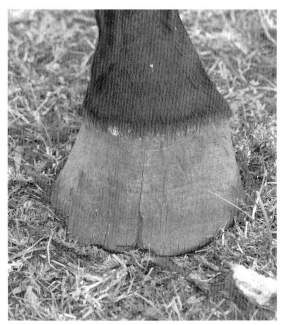

Figure 4.15 *Overlong foot showing cracking and spreading of the hoof wall*

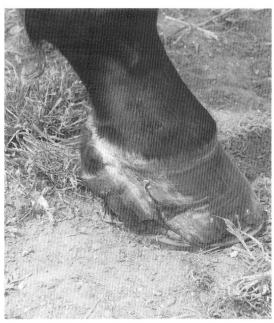

Figure 4.16 *Cracking and deformity of the hoof wall due to an old injury to the coronary band*

- injury to the coronary band (*Figures 4.16 and 4.17*) or foot, e.g. an overreach, brushing injury, or direct blow to the hoof
- thin walls
- dry brittle horn.

Clinical signs

When the crack is superficial and does not involve the sensitive tissues, the horse remains sound.

Lameness occurs if the sensitive laminae are pinched by movement of the hoof wall or if the underlying sensitive tissues become infected. In these cases, pus may exude from the base of the crack.

Treatment

For all hoof wall cracks:
- trim the hoof to a normal shape

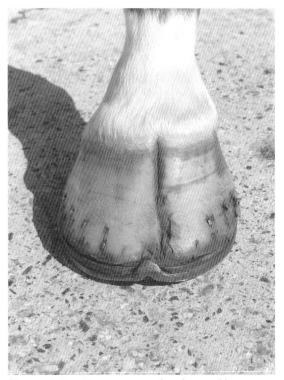

Figure 4.17 *Permanent sandcrack caused by a coronary band injury*

- shoe the horse to minimise the movement of the wall on either side of the crack
- supplement the diet with biotin and methionine or MSM to improve the quality of horn
- make sure the feet do not become excessively dry.

Superficial sandcracks

A nail or toe clip positioned on either side of the crack is usually all that is required to stabilise the hoof wall.

The crack normally grows out at a rate of 6–10 mm a month. However, if the coronary band is permanently damaged, corrective shoeing must be continued for the rest of the horse's life.

Grasscracks

A horizontal bar, or triangle and bar design, is grooved at the upper limit of the crack to prevent it extending towards the coronary band (*Figure 4.18*).

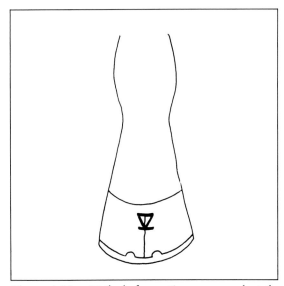

Figure 4.18 *Method of correcting a grasscrack at the toe*

The grooves should be 2 cm in length and go through the entire thickness of the wall to the white line.

Toe clips are then positioned on either side of the crack to prevent spreading of the hoof wall.

Deep infected cracks

If the crack is deep and infection is present, the hoof must be thoroughly cleaned and poulticed. In some cases the crack needs to be widened to expose the infected tissues and establish drainage.

Once the infection has been eliminated, the vet or farrier may drill holes through the hoof wall on either side of the crack and 'lace' it up using umbilical tape or stainless steel wire. The crack is then filled with an acrylic resin to prevent the entry of dirt. This stabilises the hoof wall.

Whenever a hoof injury occurs, check that the horse is protected against tetanus.

Thrush

Thrush is an infection which affects the frog.

The horn decomposes and forms black material which collects in the clefts and has a characteristic and unpleasant smell.

If left untreated, the infection can penetrate the underlying sensitive tissues and cause lameness.

Treatment

1) The foot must be thoroughly cleaned using water and a stiff brush. An old dandy brush is ideal for this purpose. Spe-

cial attention should be paid to the clefts of the frog to ensure removal of all the debris.

2) Any loose pieces of frog should be trimmed by the farrier as they can trap infection in the clefts.

3) Thrush recognised in the early stages may be treated in one of several ways. The daily scrubbing is followed by application of:
   - a spray containing gentian violet and an antibiotic, or
   - a mixture made up of equal parts of phenol, 10 per cent formalin and iodine, or
   - Stockholm tar.

4) If infection has entered the sensitive tissues, the foot must be poulticed.

5) The horse should be stabled on clean dry bedding or turned out into a dry field.

Prevention

Thrush is caused by poor foot care and a lack of stable hygiene. To prevent the disease:
- pick the feet out at least once daily
- make sure the bedding is clean and dry
- have the feet trimmed regularly by the farrier.

Corns

A corn is a bruise which develops on the sole in the angle between the wall and the bars.

Causes

Corns usually occur on the inner aspect of the horse's front feet.

They are caused by:
- leaving the shoes on too long. As the horn grows, the heels of the shoe move inside the hoof wall and press on the seat of corn (*Figure 4.19*)
- using shoes that are too small
- unbalanced feet: caused by uneven trimming or the use of a single road stud. The heel on the raised side is subjected to increased concussion as the foot contacts the ground
- poor hoof conformation: flat feet and low heels predispose to corns.

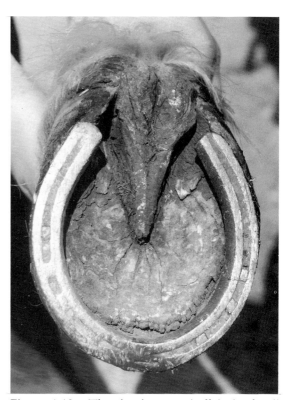

Figure 4.19   *This shoe has moved off the hoof wall and is pressing on the seat of corn*

Clinical signs

- Lameness may be slight or severe. It is usually accentuated by turning or working

on a circle with the affected foot on the inside.
- the horse reacts to hoof testers applied to the seat of corn
- when the shoe is removed and the horn lightly pared, a red area of bruising is usually visible.

Treatment

The area of discoloured horn is pared by the farrier or vet, to relieve the pressure.

Tubbing or poulticing is recommended twice daily until the horse is sound.

If the corn has become infected and pus is released, the treatment is as described for pus in the foot (see earlier in this chapter).

The horse must be rested and not reshod until completely sound.

Before shoeing, the affected area of hoof should be hardened with a gentian violet and antibiotic spray or a mixture of phenol, formalin and iodine obtained from the vet. Care should be taken to avoid further bruising as the condition may recur and can become chronic. It may be necessary to have the shoes replaced every four weeks.

Bruised Soles

Bruised soles are a common problem in horses with thin soles and flat feet.

Causes

The causes include:
- treading on a stone or other sharp object
- concussion from working on hard or uneven ground

- incorrectly fitted shoes
- unbalanced feet.

Clinical signs

Horses show differing degrees of lameness. These include:
- sudden acute lameness
- lameness for one or two strides after treading on a stone, then continuing normally. The next day the horse comes out of the box lame
- slight or no lameness on a soft surface. The lameness is accentuated on hard or uneven ground.

Other signs include:
- withdrawal of the foot when the bruised area is squeezed with hoof testers
- red areas of bruised horn on the sole of white feet.

Treatment

Box rest the horse and provide a clean, deep bed. If necessary, remove the shoe.

Poultice the foot for two days and then commence tubbing twice daily until sound. A bad bruise may take up to three weeks to resolve.

In severe cases, anti-inflammatory drugs such as phenylbutazone may be prescribed.

The sole should be hardened before the horse is turned out or resumes work. This is especially important when the foot is still soft from poulticing. It can be achieved by regular applications of a gentian violet and antibiotic spray or a phenol, iodine and formalin mixture.

A protective pad may be fitted to protect the sole when the shoe is replaced. As soon as the condition has resolved, the pad should be removed for the following reasons:
- the sole sweats under a pad, making the horn soft and susceptible to thrush infection

- mud and small stones can become trapped between the pad and the shoe
- shoes are harder to fit and tend to pull off more readily when pads are used.

A wide-webbed shoe that is seated out can be used as an alternative to pads to protect thin or recently bruised soles (*Figures 4.20 and 4.21*).

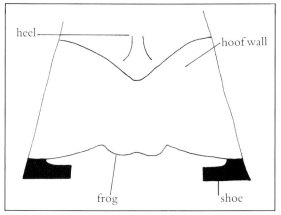

Figure 4.20   *Hind view of a foot showing a wide web seated-out shoe. This protects the sole without subjecting it to any pressure*

Occasionally a bruised sole becomes infected and develops into an abscess. The horse becomes acutely lame and the vet or farrier must be called.

Long Toes and Collapsed Heels

These are common faults of hoof conformation in the shod horse (*Figure 4.22*).

Causes

They are caused by infrequent or incorrect trimming – the toes are allowed to grow too

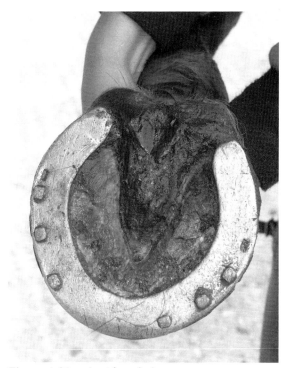

Figure 4.21   *A wide web shoe*

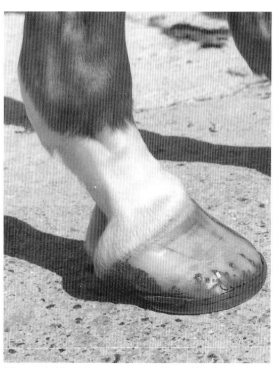

Figure 4.22   *Long toes and collapsed heels*

long and the heels become too low. As a result, the horse's weight is shifted backwards onto the heels instead of being uniformly distributed around the hoof wall. The wall at the heels may not be strong enough to support the additional weight and the following changes occur.

Clinical signs

- The quarters spread
- The heels collapse forwards under the foot
- The pastern/hoof axis is broken because the anterior hoof wall becomes more sloping or even concave in outline
- The long toe and altered hoof angle impose a strain on the sensitive laminae attaching the hoof wall to the pedal bone. The laminae at the toe may become torn and bruised, causing lameness
- The long toe, low heel conformation puts abnormal strain on the flexor tendons and accessory (check) ligament.

Treatment

Correction takes 1–2 years.

During this time the feet must be trimmed and shod at intervals of 4–6 weeks. The toe is cut back as far as possible but very little horn is removed from the heels.

Two methods of shoeing are popular for correction of this condition.

- Shoes may be fitted wide at the heels with the branches extending slightly beyond the ground surface of the foot. This increases the bearing surface and when combined with corrective trimming, restores a more normal distribution of the horse's weight
- The eggbar shoe (*Figure 4.23*) is also used to increase the area of ground contact and support the weight of the horse.

Both types of shoe encourage the new horn to grow down in the correct direction.

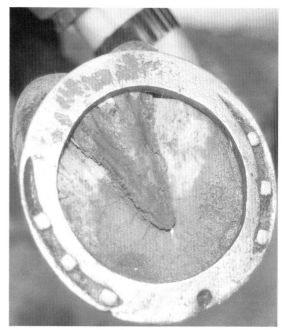

Figure 4.23   *An eggbar shoe*

Horn growth should be stimulated by using the measures discussed for brittle feet (see earlier in this chapter).

Laminitis

Laminitis is a painful condition where circulatory changes cause inflammation and congestion of the sensitive laminae of the feet.

Although it most commonly affects overweight ponies and show horses, laminitis can affect any type of horse at any time of year.

The course of the disease

The condition is not fully understood.

A number of factors cause the animal's blood pressure to rise and this increases the blood supply to the feet. The blood, however, is shunted from the small arteries directly to the veins with a reduced flow through the capillary beds supplying the sensitive laminae. Blood clots sometimes form and further impair the circulation.

As the sensitive laminae are deprived of their oxygen and nutrient supply, they become inflamed and swollen. Fluid leaks from the blood vessels and the increased pressure inside the hoof causes intense pain.

In severe cases, haemorrhage and exudate from the inflamed laminae may build up sufficient pressure to escape at the coronary band.

Rotation of the pedal bone

Unless the cause is removed and treatment is started immediately, the sensitive laminae begin to die.

Approximately 600 of these sensitive laminae hold the pedal bone in position by interdigitating with a corresponding number of insensitive laminae in the hoof capsule. Once this attachment is weakened, the upward pull from the deep digital flexor tendon plus the weight of the horse cause a rotation and/or sinking of the pedal bone within the hoof. The sole becomes flattened or convex to accommodate its new position. The blood vessels between the sole and the pedal bone become compressed (*Figure 4.24*).

Ultimately, the toe of the pedal bone may penetrate the sole in front of the point of the frog. In acute cases, this can happen very quickly.

Causes

A number of different factors can cause laminitis. Animals that are overweight or have suffered previous attacks are particularly susceptible.

The causes include:
- access to *lush* or *fast growing (e.g. recently fertilized) grass* or *clover*
- eating *large quantities of feed*
- *toxaemia* from any condition where bacterial toxins are absorbed, e.g. retained placenta, severe colic or diarrhoea
- *concussion* from fast or prolonged exercise on hard ground
- *irregular or incorrect hoof trimming*
- *excessive weight-bearing on one limb*, e.g. with a fracture or severe tendon strain, the uninjured, supporting leg may develop laminitis
- *stress*, e.g. frequent travelling of overweight show animals

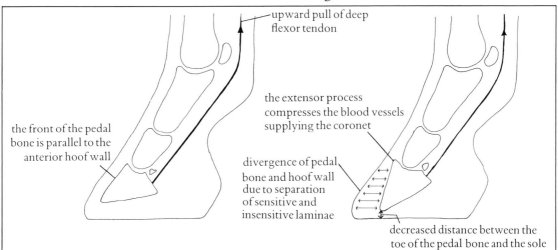

Figure 4.24   *Position of the pedal bone:* (left) *normal;* (right) *rotated pedal bone*

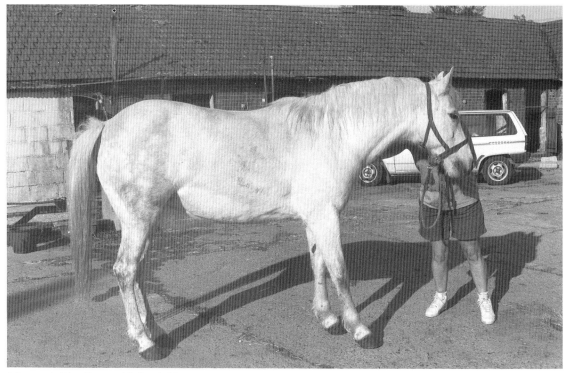

Figure 4.25 *Pony with laminitis*

- *corticosteroids* can cause rotation of the pedal bone in susceptible animals
- *pituitary gland tumours* in old ponies may cause laminitis.

Clinical signs

Any number of feet may be affected, but the condition most commonly involves the two front feet.

The following symptoms may be observed:

Stance

Many laminitic animals adopt a characteristic stance. The forelegs are stretched forwards and most of the weight is borne on the heels; this takes the pressure off the toe. The hind limbs are positioned well forward under the body (*Figure 4.25*). In severe cases, the animal may spend much of the time lying flat out on its side. When standing, the weight is constantly shifted from one foot to another.

Reluctance to move

Laminitic horses and ponies are reluctant to move.

When forced to walk, they take careful, 'pottery' strides; this is exaggerated when turning. They often resist when asked to lift a foot and if forced to stand on three legs, may collapse.

Heat

The coronary band may be abnormally warm, but this is an unreliable sign.

Reaction to hoof testers

The sole is abnormally sensitive to pressure. Hoof testers cause affected animals to flinch when applied to the area just in front of the point of the frog.

Pulse, respiration and temperature

With intense pain, the pulse and respiration rates increase, and some animals have a temperature. They may tremble and appear anxious.

An abnormally strong pulse can often be palpated where the digital artery runs over the fetlock.

Mild or chronic cases

These animals may show some or all of the following signs:
- intermittent lameness on hard or uneven ground
- apparent stiffness rather than obvious lameness when both front feet are affected
- laminitic rings and a distorted hoof shape
- sensitivity to hoof testers applied between the point of the frog and the toe.

Effects on hoof growth and conformation

The effects of laminitis on hoof growth and conformation may include:

Coronary band depression

An abnormal depression may be palpated on the front of the coronary band if the pedal bone has started to move.

Growth rings on the hoof wall

As the pedal bone rotates, its extensor process compresses the blood supply to the coronet. This slows down the rate of new horn production at the toe.

The result is laminitic growth rings which are wider at the heel than the toe (*Figure 4.26*).

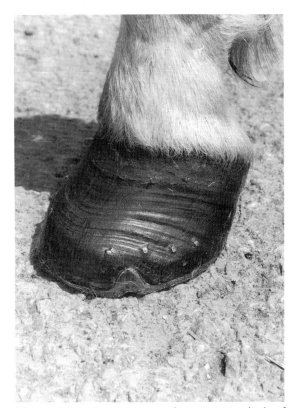

Figure 4.26   *Laminitic growth rings. Note the hoof has high heels and a long toe*

The hoof changes shape, developing high heels and a long toe with a concave anterior hoof wall.

White line

With chronic cases, the movement of the pedal bone is less drastic but inflammation causes the production of excessive amounts of horny tissue between the outer hoof wall and the sensitive laminae. This widens the white line at the ground surface. It becomes an area of weakness and makes the horse susceptible to abscesses and seedy toe.

Sole

The sole may drop, becoming flat or convex.

Treatment

Laminitis should be regarded as an emergency since prompt treatment can make a significant difference to the outcome of the case.
    The aims of treatment are:
- relief of pain
- restoration of normal circulation in the foot
- stabilisation of the pedal bone within the hoof.

Medical treatment

The vet may prescribe some of the following treatments:
- *Phenylbutazone* – for its analgesic and anti-inflammatory properties.
- *Flunixin meglumine* – for analgesia and protection against bacterial toxins.
- *ACP* – to calm an anxious horse and lower the blood pressure.
- *Antibiotics* – if toxaemia is suspected as the cause.
- *Liquid paraffin* – given by stomach tube, if large quantities of grain have been ingested.
- *Probiotics* – to help restore the normal microbial population of the gut.
- *Vasodilators* – e.g. isoxuprine, may be

given to encourage blood flow through the foot. Their value is as yet undetermined.

Management and nursing

Stabling

The animal should be stabled at the start of treatment. As its condition improves it may be allowed access to a smooth concrete yard or a small starvation paddock with no grass.

Bedding

Provide a deep bed of clean shavings, sand or peat. These materials conform to the shape of the foot and give some support and comfort.

Feeding

Do not feed concentrates or allow grazing. Divide the hay ration into three small feeds.
    Avoid drastic starvation or the pony may develop hyperlipaemia.
    If your mare is in foal or you are not sure how much to feed, seek veterinary advice.

Supplements

The diet can be supplemented with substances to improve the growth rate and quality of horn. Examples include:
- biotin and methionine
- MSM (methyl-sulphonyl-methane)
- multi-component mixes.

Exercise

Exercise is *harmful* if the pedal bone is rotating or sinking. Forcing the horse to walk causes further separation of the weakened laminae.

In cases where the pedal bone is stable, short periods of walking on soft ground encourages circulation in the feet; 10 minutes every two hours is recommended.

If, at any stage, exercise makes the feet more painful, *do not continue* as the pedal bone may be starting to move.

Bathing

Hot or cold bathing is unlikely to make any real difference to the outcome of the case.

Warm water bathing of the feet dilates the arterioles and increases the blood supply.

Cold water treatment can give temporary pain relief but it constricts the blood vessels which is undesirable.

Hoof care

Where laminitis is confirmed, the feet require immediate attention and careful monitoring.

Removal of shoes

Whether or not the shoes are removed depends on the severity of the case and the condition of the feet.

Where the sole has dropped, the horse will be more comfortable wearing shoes.

Frog support

The vet will tape a triangular pad or roll of bandage over the frog. This is a temporary measure to provide support and increase the horse's comfort until radiography and corrective farriery can be arranged.

Corrective trimming and shoeing

The long-term aim of corrective trimming and shoeing is to restore the normal alignment of the pedal bone and hoof capsule. The vet and the farrier work together. Trimming is usually carried out at monthly intervals (*Figure 4.27*).

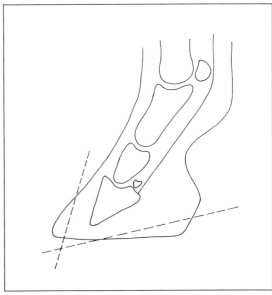

Figure 4.27 *Diagram to show how corrective trimming can realign the pedal bone and hoof wall*

X-rays are taken at the start of treatment and at regular intervals to check on the progress. After several months of careful trimming, many ponies become sound and are able to resume normal work.

Using the x-rays as a guide, the farrier will:
- shorten long toes
- rasp back the front of the hoof wall until it is parallel with the pedal bone
- remove excessive heel growth. In acute cases, the heels are lowered gradually or the sudden increase in tension on the deep digital flexor tendon could rotate the pedal bone.
- fit corrective shoes where required.

Special techniques

These are used to try and stabilise the pedal bone when it is sinking or rotating.

Use of heart bar shoes

The shoe is designed to provide support to the pedal bone through the frog, without interfering with the blood supply to the sole.

X-rays are taken with markers to show the position of the coronary band, the anterior hoof wall and a point 1 cm behind the point of the frog (*Figure 4.28*). These are essential for correct fitting of the shoe which can otherwise cause serious and irreversible damage.

Glue-on shoes are often used to eliminate the pain and concussion experienced by laminitic ponies when conventional shoes are nailed in place.

The shoes are replaced at monthly intervals.

Dorsal wall resection

This involves removal of the front of the hoof wall. The aims of the procedure are to:

- remove the pressure from the blood vessels supplying the coronary band
- allow inflammatory exudate to escape, relieving pressure and pain
- allow the new hoof wall to grow parallel to the front of the pedal bone
- encourage realignment of the pedal bone when combined with frog support.

Cutting the deep digital flexor tendon

With longstanding rotation, the deep digital flexor tendon shortens and is unable to stretch to allow repositioning of the pedal bone. Cutting this tendon permits realignment, but the horse will not be sound enough to work again.

Prognosis

With prompt treatment and good management, many mild cases make a good recovery within a few days and no specialist treatment is required. However, when the pedal bone has changed position or the feet are misshapen, corrective trimming is required for many months.

Figure 4.28 *Radiograph with markers showing rotation of the pedal bone*

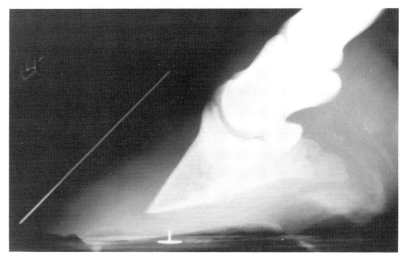

When serious changes have occurred in the foot, the commitment of the owner must be 100 per cent before embarking upon a long term correction programme. The management of these animals is time-consuming, expensive and, at times, disappointing.

In some cases, the suffering of the animal is so intense that euthanasia is the only course of action.

Prevention

Laminitis can usually be prevented by sensible management.
- Restrict grazing when the pasture is lush or the grass is growing quickly. This is especially important with overweight or susceptible animals. Most ponies are safe if allowed to graze for an hour in the morning and evening.
- If necessary, use a starvation paddock. This is easily made with an electric fence. Alternatively, fit a muzzle to restrict grazing while still allowing the pony to exercise and drink
- Ensure the feet are regularly trimmed and shod
- Avoid trotting on the road and on hard ground
- Keep the feedroom locked
- Ensure prompt treatment of conditions such as retained placenta and colic.

Seedy Toe

Seedy toe is a condition where the sensitive and insensitive laminae separate at the white line, allowing a cavity to form (*Figure 4.29*). This is filled by weak, crumbly horn.

The separation is widest near the ground surface and narrows towards the coronet.

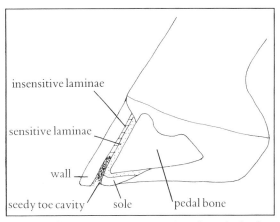

Figure 4.29   *Diagrammatic section through the foot showing a seedy toe cavity*

The cavity may be shallow or deep. If it becomes packed with soil and other foreign material, secondary infection may develop.

Causes

The causes are not fully understood. The condition is a common sequel to laminitis.

Clinical signs

Many horses show no symptoms and the problem is discovered and dealt with by the farrier.

Lameness occurs if:
- secondary infection develops
- a large area is involved so the weight of the horse is supported by a considerably reduced number of laminae which then become inflamed.

Treatment

1) Long toes should be trimmed as they encourage separation of the sensitive and insensitive laminae.

2) When there is just a small cavity, the crumbly horn is removed and the hole should be packed with cotton wool and Stockholm tar. Deeper cavities must be scrubbed clean and thoroughly dried. To prevent them refilling with debris, they can be packed as above or filled by the farrier or vet with substances that set to the shape of the cavity.

   A broad-webbed shoe is fitted to protect the area and hold the dressing in place.

3) When the cavity is too deep and narrow to allow proper cleaning, the overlying hoof wall may be removed by the farrier or vet.

   New horn will grow down at a rate of approximately 1 cm a month.

4) If infection is present, the shoe is not replaced. The foot should be tubbed and poulticed twice a day. Warm magnesium sulphate paste is effective at drawing infection from these awkward cavities.

The defect grows out over a period of time. Affected horses suffer fewer setbacks if the feet are kept clean and dry.

Supplementing the diet with biotin and methionine or MSM encourages the growth of healthy horn.

Fracture of the Pedal Bone

Fractures of the horse's pedal bone are not uncommon; they usually occur in the fore feet.

Causes

- Trauma, e.g. landing on a hard, uneven surface or kicking a solid wall.

- Foreign body penetration.
- Infection.

Clinical signs

- Sudden onset of acute lameness.
- Heat in the foot and coronary band.
- Increased ditigal pulse.
- Pain when hoof testers are applied.

Diagnosis

The diagnosis needs to be confirmed by radiography.

A hairline fracture may not show up on the x-rays for at least two weeks after the injury has occurred. The vet may have to take several views of the foot on more than one occasion in order to confirm the diagnosis.

Treatment

Treatment is either conservative or surgical. The aim is to stop any movement occurring between the fractured edges of bone.

Conservative treatment

A bar shoe with quarter clips is fitted every 4–6 weeks for at least six months. This type of shoe prevents expansion of the hoof wall at the quarters and helps to stabilise the fracture.

A period of three months complete box rest should be followed by three months of confinement to a small paddock or yard.

The horse will require a total of 6–12 months off work.

Surgical treatment

If the fracture extends to the articular surface

of the coffin joint, it should be stabilised by screwing the two bone fragments together. The screw stops movement between the fragments and reduces the risk of degenerative joint disease.

The subsequent management is as described for conservative treatment.

Prognosis

The prognosis for pedal bone fractures that do not extend into the coffin joint is good.

If the joint is involved, the prognosis is grave.

Sidebone

Sidebone is ossification of the cartilages which are attached to the pedal bone (*Figure 4.30*).

These cartilages can be palpated above the coronary band towards the back of the foot.

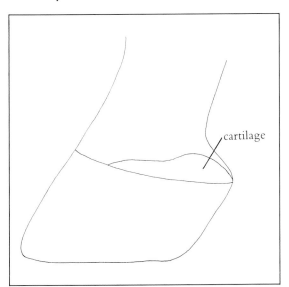

Figure 4.30   *The position of the cartilages of the foot*

They are normally quite springy, but feel hard and unyielding when a horse has sidebone.

The condition is most common in the front feet. It is rarely a cause of lameness; many sound horses have sidebone.

Causes

- Concussion.
  This may be accentuated by:
  – foot imbalance
  – poor conformation, e.g. horses that are 'base-narrow, toe-in' tend to develop lateral sidebone. Those that have 'base-wide, toe-out' conformation may develop sidebone on the medial side
- Direct injuries to the cartilages of the feet.

Clinical signs

When these occur:
- the horse is lame; there may be some shortening of the stride while the new bone is forming
- pressing the affected cartilage causes pain during the active phase
- fracture of a large sidebone causes acute lameness.

As soon as the inflammation has subsided there are no further symptoms.

Treatment

No treatment is required in the majority of cases.
- When one side is affected more than the other, the balance of the foot should be checked and corrected if necessary
- Box rest is required where heat and pain are present
- Fractures heal with 12 weeks box rest

- Occasionally a small fragment of bone has to be surgically removed

Navicular Disease

Navicular disease is a progressive, degenerative condition involving the navicular bone, the navicular bursa and the deep digital flexor tendon. It affects one, or more commonly, both front feet.

The disease is seen in all types of horse, but rarely affects ponies. Performance horses engaged in seasonal work seem particularly susceptible. The symptoms usually develop when the horse is 6–12 years old.

Navicular disease is less common than is generally believed. It is discussed in detail because of the concern it generates amongst horse owners and prospective purchasers.

Causes

The cause of navicular disease is uncertain. One popular view is that poor drainage of blood from the foot leads to:
- a rise in blood pressure within the bone
- formation of blood clots in the arteries supplying the navicular bone
- thickening of the artery walls.

This reduces the blood flow through the foot, which is also impaired by factors such as poor hoof conformation, enforced rest and irregular work.

The reduced blood supply leads to inadequate nutrition of the bone and degenerative changes begin.

Other suggested causes include:
- concussion
- excessive tension from the suspensory ligaments that attach the navicular bone to the long pastern
- abnormal mechanical compression of the bone in horses with 'long toe, low heel' conformation.

The picture is far from clear.

Changes in the navicular bone

Ulcers develop in the smooth cartilage layer covering the back of the navicular bone. In places the cartilage is completely eroded and the bone becomes exposed. This results in continual trauma to the deep digital flexor tendon.

In advanced cases of navicular disease, adhesions form between the tendon and the navicular bone.

The pain associated with the disease is attributed to:
- elevation of blood pressure within the bone
- trauma to the deep digital flexor tendon.

Clinical signs

Change in action

Over a period of time, there is a gradual shortening of the horse's stride.

The toe is placed on the ground first to reduce concussion at the heel. This gives a 'pottery' gait and the horse tends to trip and stumble.

Lameness

Navicular disease is insidious in onset and rarely causes sudden lameness. In the early stages, the lameness is slight and intermittent, tending to improve with exercise. It is most obvious when the horse works on a circle, especially when lunged at trot on a hard, flat surface.

Symptoms observed at rest

These include:
- shifting the weight from one foot to the other
- standing with one foot in front of the other with the heel slightly raised. This relieves the pressure between the deep digital flexor tendon and the navicular bone and is known as 'pointing' (*Figure 4.31*). When both feet are painful, the feet are alternately pointed
- digging a hole in the bed and standing with the toes in the hole and the heels raised on the edge
- contraction of the heels as the disease progresses may cause the hoof to become upright and boxy. When only one foot is affected, the two front feet become dissimilar in size and shape.

Diagnosis

Diagnosis is made on the clinical signs, nerve blocks and radiography.

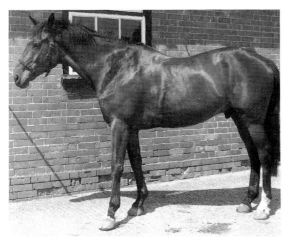

Figure 4.31   *Horse with navicular disease, 'pointing' the left fore foot*

The lameness is usually eliminated by a nerve block which desensitises the back of the foot.

When the pain is removed from the obviously lame foot, the horse often goes lame on the opposite leg. This is because the condition is usually bilateral, but more advanced in one limb than the other.

When the navicular regions of both feet are desensitised, the horse often becomes sound.

Radiographic changes

On an x-ray of a normal navicular bone, 5–7 dark cone-shaped areas can be seen on the lower edge of the bone (*Figure 4.32*). These are channels where arteries enter the bone; they are called 'nutrient foramina'.

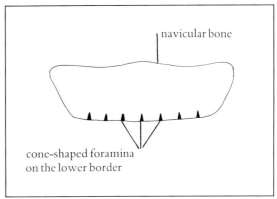

Figure 4.32   *The outline of a normal navicular bone*

Changes which may occur in navicular disease include:
- an increase in number or alteration in size and shape of foramina (*Figures 4.33 and 4.34*) as more blood vessels develop to nourish the damaged bone
- the development of any foramina on the wings or upper border of the bone
- increased density of bone around the foramina
- a cyst-like lesion in the centre of the bone.

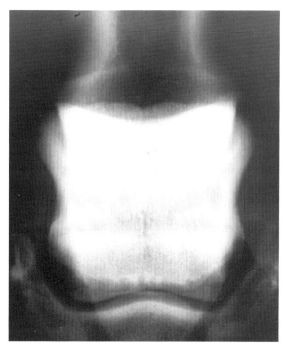

Figure 4.33   *Radiograph showing navicular disease*

Interpretation of the x-rays is not always easy, as many sound horses have some changes within their navicular bones.

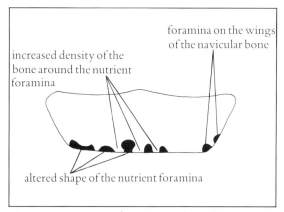

increased density of the bone around the nutrient foramina

foramina on the wings of the navicular bone

altered shape of the nutrient foramina

Figure 4.34   *Line drawing to show the abnormal changes seen on the radiograph in* Figure 4.33

Treatment

The earlier treatment begins, the greater the chance of prolonging the horse's working life.

Current treatments include:

1) Corrective farriery

This is an essential part of any treatment programme.

The foot must be balanced. It should be trimmed to establish and maintain a straight pastern/hoof axis. Where necessary, the toe is shortened.

Growth and expansion of the heel should be encouraged by fitting the shoe wide at the heels. Eggbar shoes are recommended for horses with collapsed heels.

In advanced cases, the pressure on the deep digital flexor tendon can be relieved by raising the heels. This may improve the horse's gait but is not generally recommended as it can cause other problems (e.g. contraction of the heels) in the long term.

2) Exercise

Exercise is necessary for the normal flow of blood through the foot. If possible, the horse should be turned out to encourage continuous, gentle exercise.

3) Isoxuprine

Isoxuprine is a drug which improves blood flow through the foot by dilating the arteries. It is administered orally. Some horses improve or become sound after a course of treatment.

4) Warfarin

Warfarin prolongs the clotting time of blood and reduces the likelihood of further clots forming in the arteries. It also reduces the viscosity of blood so it flows more easily through the damaged vessels.

Warfarin is a drug that must be used with care. The clotting time of the blood must be closely monitored to reduce the risk of serious haemorrhage. It is not compatible with many other drugs.

5) Non-steroidal anti-inflammatory drugs

These drugs may alleviate the pain but do not halt the progress of the disease.

6) Navicular suspensory desmotomy

The suspensory ligaments joining the upper border of the navicular bone to the long pastern are cut under general anaesthesia. This reduces the stress on the navicular bone as the limb bears weight. In some cases the operation reduces or eliminates the lameness.

7) Neurectomy

Part of the nerve supplying sensation to the back of the foot is removed. This results in desensitisation of the area around the navicular bone and many horses improve or become sound.

The nerve can regrow, however, and there are complications associated with this operation. They include:
- formation of a painful swelling (neuroma) at the cut end of the nerve
- rupture of the deep digital flexor tendon. This occurs if adhesions have developed between the navicular bone and the deep digital flexor tendon. When the pain is removed and the horse starts to adopt a normal gait, the adhesions are torn and the weakened tendon may rupture.

Prognosis

At this time, there is no cure for navicular disease.

By the time the horse is lame and radiographic changes are visible, the disease is well established.

Owing to the constant pressure between the navicular bone and the deep digital flexor tendon, the lesions are unlikely to heal. At best, the treatments available slow down the degenerative changes or make the horse more comfortable.

The prognosis is therefore extremely guarded.

Pedal Ostitis

Pedal ostitis is inflammation of the pedal bone.

Causes

Inflammation may occur as a result of long-term concussion and chronic bruising of the sole.

Horses with flat feet or thin soles that work on hard or rough ground are particularly susceptible.

Alternatively, pedal ostitis may develop secondary to other foot problems such as laminitis, puncture wounds or persistent corns.

Clinical signs

The disease usually affects both front feet. In the early stages, the horse works normally on

soft ground but shortens its stride on hard surfaces.
- this progresses to lameness when worked on hard ground
- the lameness improves with rest but recurs when work is resumed
- pain may be present when hoof testers are applied, but this is an unreliable sign.

X-ray findings

In the past, pedal ostitis has been overdiagnosed as the cause of lameness on the basis of x-ray findings.

The radiographic features include:
- an irregular outline to the bone
- loss of bone density
- increased width and number of vascular channels
- new bone formation.

However, with the exception of the last feature, these variations are regularly found on x-rays of sound horses. A diagnosis of pedal ostitis can only be made if there are marked radiographic changes and other causes of foot lameness have been excluded. Even then, the diagnosis is impossible to prove as there is no nerve block that specifically desensitises the pedal bone.

Treatment and prognosis

Where there is extensive deposition of new bone or a considerable loss of bone density, there is no effective treatment and the prognosis is poor.

In less severe cases, the horse will benefit from:
- a period of rest
- fitting of wide-webbed shoes seated out to protect the sole
- application of a phenol, iodine and formalin mixture to harden soft or thin soles
- modification of the exercise programme to avoid working on hard or stony ground.

5 Joint Problems

Synovial Joints

Horses experience a wide range of joint problems. Most of these conditions involve synovial joints (*Figure 5.1*), e.g. the fetlock, knee and hock.

Structure of a synovial joint

The joint capsule is composed of two layers:
- an outer fibrous layer, which is attached to the periosteum of the bone
- an inner synovial membrane which secretes synovial fluid. This nourishes the articular cartilage and has a lubricating role within the joint.

The articular surfaces of the bones are covered with smooth cartilage.

Joint disease

Joint disease can lead to lameness or permanent loss of use, so early diagnosis and treatment is essential. Examples include sprains, infection and degenerative joint disease (arthritis).

Sprains

A sprain occurs when the fibres of the joint capsule or the supporting ligaments are torn.

Causes

It is usually the result of a twist or wrench when the horse slips or works on uneven ground.

It may be mild with just a few torn fibres,

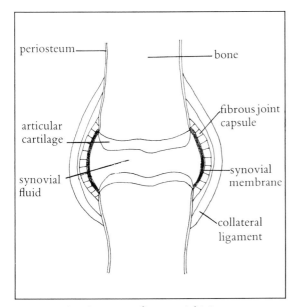

Figure 5.1   *Structure of a synovial joint*

or severe with considerable haemorrhage and rupture of a ligament.

Clinical signs

The symptoms are similar, regardless of which joint is affected.

There is:
- lameness
- heat
- distension of the joint capsule due to increased production of synovial fluid
- soft tissue swelling around the joint
- pain and increased lameness when the joint is flexed.

Treatment

Treatment is likely to include:
- cold therapy for the first 48 hours
- support bandaging where practical
- non-steroidal anti-inflammatory drugs, e.g. phenylbutazone
- box rest.

The period of rest depends on the severity of the sprain. As the injury heals, short periods of walking in hand are introduced.

With severe sprains, injection of sodium hyaluronate into the joint space aids recovery. This treatment is very expensive.

Ultrasound, laser or magnetic field therapy may also be beneficial.

If the lameness persists for more than two weeks, x-rays should be taken to see if there are any bony changes at the site where the joint capsule or ligaments attach to the bone.

Prognosis

If the horse is adequately rested and there is no major damage to the collateral ligaments, the prognosis is good.

Joint Infection

Bacterial infection of a joint can very quickly cause cartilage destruction and the development of infectious arthritis.

Causes

- Bacteria may enter a joint from a penetrating wound.
- In young foals, bacteria from the gut or an infected navel may be carried in the blood and localise in one or more joints. This gives rise to the condition known as joint-ill.
- Occasionally a joint becomes infected following an intra-articular injection.

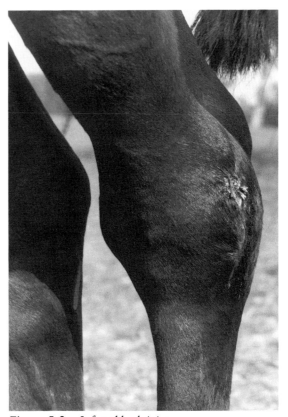

Figure 5.2   *Infected hock joint*

Clinical signs

- Sudden onset of severe lameness.
- Distension of the joint capsule (*Figure 5.2*).
- Pain when the joint is touched or flexed.

Other symptoms which may occur include:
- increased temperature
- depression
- loss of appetite.

Diagnosis

Diagnosis is made on:
- clinical signs
- the changed appearance and composition of synovial fluid. Fluid withdrawn from infected joints looks cloudy and has a very high white cell count.
- radiography.

    The radiographic changes include:
    - alterations in the width of the joint spaces
    - destruction of bone
    - proliferation of new bone.

Treatment

Joint infection is an emergency and treatment should commence as soon as the condition is suspected.
    Treatment includes:
- broad-spectrum antibiotics, administered for up to 4–6 weeks
- draining and flushing of the joint with several litres of saline to remove enzymes and other substances that are harmful to articular cartilage
- analgesics.

The horse will then require a long period of rest.

Prognosis

Unless aggressive treatment is started immediately, the prognosis is poor. In some cases the horse appears to recover, then the infection flares up again.

Degenerative Joint Disease

Degenerative joint disease is a disease of the articular cartilage within a joint. Examples include bone spavin and ringbone.

Causes

It may develop rapidly following:
- a severe sprain
- a fracture
- infection.

It can also develop over a longer period of time as a result of chronic, low-grade strains imposed by poor conformation and normal work.

The course of the disease

Inflammation of the joint capsule leads to production of enzymes and prostaglandins which break down the articular cartilage, causing it to become thin and ulcerated.
    Spurs of new bone may develop around the joint and bony deposits form within the joint capsule and associated ligaments.
    As the disease progresses, the joint space may become completely filled by new bone.

Occasionally the bones fuse together and are incapable of further movement.

Clinical signs

These are variable depending on the cause of the problem and the joint(s) affected. They include:
- heat
- distension of the joint capsule due to increased synovial fluid production
- soft tissue swelling around the joint
- lameness, which may be gradual or sudden in onset
- pain on flexion of the joint
- increased lameness following flexion.

In advanced cases there is:
- joint enlargement due to fibrous tissue and new bone production
- a reduced range of joint movement.

Diagnosis

Diagnosis is made on:

1) Clinical signs

2) Radiography

The radiographic signs include:
- periosteal bone proliferation
- spurs of new bone at the joint margins
- narrowing or disappearance of the joint spaces
- changes in density of the bone directly below the joint.

However, radiography can be misleading because:
- cartilage does not show up on x-rays, so the joint may look normal despite the ex-

istence of severe erosions in the articular cartilage
- bony changes around the joint may not be the cause of the lameness – this can only be determined by nerve blocks.

3) Intra-articular anaesthesia (nerve blocks)

4) Synovial fluid examination

The composition of synovial fluid changes as degenerative joint disease progresses.

5) Arthroscopy

The articular cartilage on some joint surfaces can be inspected using an arthroscope. The instrument is inserted via a small incision with the horse under general anaesthesia.

Treatment

There is no cure for degenerative joint disease. The aims of treatment are therefore to:
- relieve pain
- reduce joint capsule and soft tissue inflammation
- stop the cartilage destruction
- encourage cartilage healing.

Treatment will vary according to the severity of the disease, the joint affected and the type of horse.
It may include:

1) Rest

Box rest is necessary when there is soft tissue swelling and acute inflammation of the joint.

However, short periods of walking exercise in hand are necessary for normal nutrition of articular cartilage.

2) Intra-articular injection

Sodium hyaluronate or polysulphated glycosaminoglycan (PSGAG) may reduce or eliminate lameness if injected into the joint in the early stages of the disease, before radiographic changes are visible.

They are most commonly used in the knee, fetlock and coffin joints. This treatment is very expensive and carries a small risk of intra-articular infection.

The benefits of each treatment are outlined below.

Sodium hyaluronate

- suppresses inflammation of the synovial membrane
- improves the lubrication of the joint
- stimulates synthesis of sodium hyaluronate by the synovial membrane.

Up to three treatments are required at seven day intervals, although in some cases a single injection can have a long-lasting result.

The horse is walked for one or two weeks following treatment, then slowly brought back into work.

Polysulphated glycosaminoglycan (PSGAG)

- PSGAG inhibits the enzymes that degrade cartilage
- stimulates the metabolism of cartilage-forming cells which play an important part in the repair process
- promotes hyaluronic acid synthesis.

When used intra-articularly, the drug is injected once a week for up to five treatments.

PSGAG can also be given intramuscularly at four day intervals for a total of seven treatments.

Once radiographic changes are present, this drug is used in preference to sodium hyaluronate.

Corticosteroids

Corticosteroids reduce inflammation of the synovial membrane and prevent the release of destructive enzymes. However, the treatment has lost its former popularity as corticosteroids are now known to have harmful effects on cartilage metabolism and healing. A temporary improvement can be followed by further degradation of the articular cartilage.

3) Non-steroidal anti-inflammatory drugs

These include phenylbutazone, flunixin meglumine and meclofenamic acid.

These drugs are anti-inflammatory and analgesic. They work by inhibiting prostaglandin synthesis by the synovial membrane.

The administration of pain-relieving drugs may extend the working life of a horse with incurable lameness. Their use should be combined with a programme of regular, light exercise. If the work is strenuous and intermittent, the joint changes may be accelerated.

4) Physiotherapy

Magnetic field therapy, for example, may improve the function of arthritic joints.

5) Topical applications

Dimethyl sulphoxide (DMSO), for example,

may be applied to reduce the soft tissue inflammation.

Prognosis

The prognosis is very guarded.

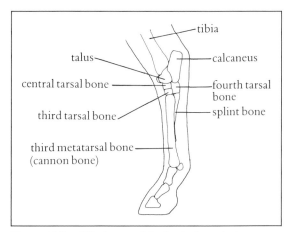

Figure 5.3 *The bones of the hock, lateral view*

Bone Spavin

Bone spavin is degenerative joint disease of the hock joint (*Figures 5.3 and 5.4*). It is a common cause of hind limb lameness.

The disease affects the distal intertarsal and the tarsometatarsal joints (*Figure 5.4*). The proximal intertarsal joint is only occasionally involved.

Causes

Constant wear and tear on the joints and ligaments make the hock susceptible to degenerative changes especially in horses that jump or make sharp turns.

Poor conformation, e.g. cow hocks or sickle hocks (*Figure 5.5*), predisposes to bone spavin.

Clinical signs

1) Gradual onset of lameness

- If both limbs are affected, the first sign is slight hind limb stiffness that wears off with exercise.
- If the horse works hard for a few days the initial stiffness may become more apparent.

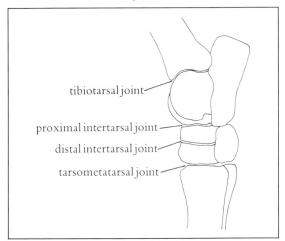

Figure 5.4 *The joints of the hock*

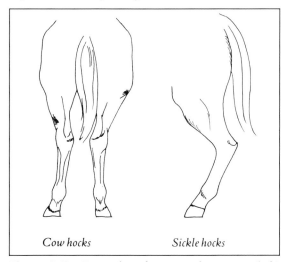

Cow hocks   *Sickle hocks*

Figure 5.5 *Examples of poor conformation:* (left) *cow hocks;* (right) *sickle hocks*

- The stiffness may also be more marked if the horse is not exercised regularly.
- Where only one limb is affected or the changes in one limb are more advanced than in the other, the horse appears unlevel or lame. This is most obvious when working on a circle.
- Jumping horses often start to refuse or jump badly.

2) Change in the hind limb action

The height of the hind foot flight arc is reduced. The hind limbs take shorter strides (do not 'track up') and the horse tends to land on its toe. The toe may be dragged, causing abnormal wear of the shoe. Irregular rhythm or occasional dragging of the toe may be heard when riding out.

3) Joint flexion

Affected horses are often uncomfortable when the hind limb is held in the flexed position for shoeing. In advanced cases flexion of the hock may be markedly reduced.

Most affected horses show a positive reaction to the spavin test. If the hock is flexed for one to one and a half minutes and the horse is trotted off on a hard flat surface, the lameness is usually accentuated for a variable number of strides. However, a negative spavin test does not exclude a diagnosis of bone spavin.

4) Swelling

A swelling may be visible on the inner aspect of the hock at the level of the distal intertarsal and tarsometatarsal joints (*Figures 5.6 and 5.7*). To check for this, stand the horse square and view the hocks from in front and behind to see if they are a matching pair. If the disease is bilateral or the horse has naturally boxy

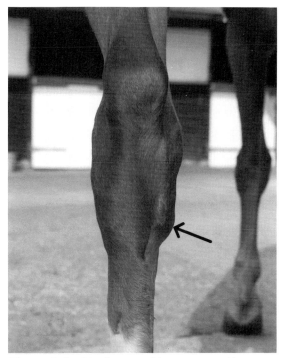

Figure 5.6 *Hind view of bone spavin (the arrow shows location)*

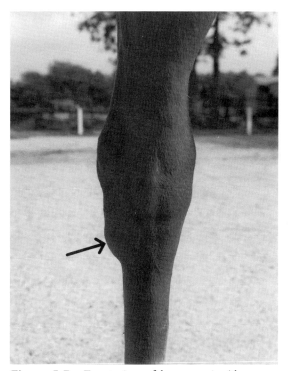

Figure 5.7 *Front view of bone spavin (the arrow shows location)*

hocks, it can be difficult to tell whether the shape is abnormal without the help of radiographs.

5) Muscle wasting

If the disease affects one hock only, there may be muscle wasting on the hindquarters of the affected side.

Diagnosis

Diagnosis is made on:
- the history
- clinical signs
- radiography. Radiographs may show:
  - a ragged appearance of the bone margins
  - spurs of new bone
  - narrowing or complete loss of the distal intertarsal and tarsometatarsal joint spaces
  - areas of reduced bone density
- nerve blocks – these are only necessary if the horse shows all the signs of spavin but the hocks appear normal on radiographs.

Treatment

Treatment is aimed at keeping the horse in work in order to accelerate fusion of the distal intertarsal and tarsometatarsal joints.

When the joint spaces have been completely replaced by bone, the horse may become sound despite some loss of hock flexibility. There is, however, no guarantee that fusion will occur and it is not possible to predict how long it will take.

1) Corrective shoeing

The toes of the hind feet should be shortened.

Shoeing with rolled toes and raised heels often improves the horse's action and comfort.

2) The use of non-steroidal anti-inflammatory drugs in conjunction with exercise

The pain may be relieved by medication, e.g. phenylbutazone, which allows the horse to continue work.

The exercise programme should be modified to include a gentle warm-up.

3) Cutting the cunean tendon

The cunean tendon runs obliquely across the inside of the hock. It may be irritated by new bone, causing pain and lameness.

Where the lameness is alleviated by infiltration of local anaesthetic around the tendon, a section may be removed. This is performed under local or general anaesthesia.

4) Arthrodesis

This procedure involves drilling out the cartilage of the distal intertarsal and tarsometatarsal joints under general anaesthesia. Occasionally the proximal intertarsal joint is included.

The aim is to hasten the fusion of the joint. The horse will need 6–12 months to recover.

Prognosis

The prognosis is guarded.

The horse may become sound enough for

light work but incapable of more demanding or competitive activities.

Ringbone

Ringbone (*Figures 5.8 and 5.9*) can occur on any of the limbs, but is more common in the forelimb. It can be subdivided into four types:

High articular (true) ringbone

This is degenerative joint disease of the pastern joint.

High non-articular (false) ringbone

New bone develops on the distal (lower) end of the long pastern and/or the proximal (up-per) end of the short pastern but does not involve the joint surface.

Low articular ringbone

This is degenerative joint disease of the coffin joint.

Low non-articular ringbone

New bone is formed on the distal end of the short pastern and/or the proximal end of the pedal bone.

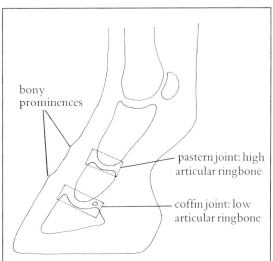

Figure 5.9   *The sites of articular ringbone*

Causes

These include:
- tearing of the periosteal attachments of:
  - collateral ligaments
  - the extensor tendon
  - the joint capsule, e.g. as the result of a sprain
- direct blows to the bone

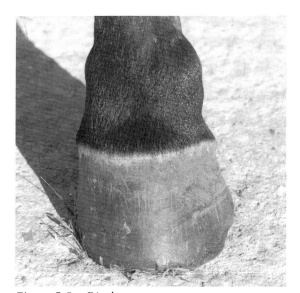

Figure 5.8   *Ringbone*

- puncture wounds and wire cuts that damage the periosteum
- poor conformation, which puts abnormal strain on one side of the limb, e.g. horses that are 'base-narrow, toe-in' are more likely to develop ringbone on the lateral side of the joint, while those with 'base-wide, toe-out' conformation may develop ringbone on the medial side
- certain types of work: e.g. articular ringbone is relatively common in polo ponies, which make sharp turns and quick stops.

Clinical signs

In most cases a hard swelling develops in the pastern region.

The degree of lameness depends on whether the joint is involved and the level of interference with soft tissue structures such as the extensor tendon.

Non-articular ringbone

There may be lameness in the early stages. When the initial inflammation has settled, the horse usually becomes sound.

Articular ringbone

Signs include:
- heat over the joint
- lameness, especially when the animal turns
- pain when the joint is flexed or twisted
- a reduced range of joint movement.

Diagnosis

Diagnosis is made on the clinical signs and is confirmed by radiography and nerve blocks.

N.B. Some horses have naturally prominent lower ends of the long pastern bone. These look like ringbone but prove to be completely normal on x-ray.

Treatment

Once ringbone has formed, very little treatment is possible.

Some horses are able to continue work with analgesics, e.g. phenylbutazone.

Occasionally the pastern joint space is completely obliterated by new bone. When the joint has fused, the horse may become sound. Fusion of the joint can also be achieved surgically.

Prognosis

The prognosis for horses with articular ringbone is guarded. It is more favourable in cases involving a hind limb.

The Stifle Joint

The stifle joint is subject to infection, strains and degenerative joint disease, but it also has the unique problem of intermittent upward fixation of the patella.

Anatomy

The stifle joint of the horse is the equivalent of the human knee. It is made up of three bones: the femur, the tibia, and the patella (kneecap) (*Figure 5.10*). The patella is attached to the tibia by the medial, middle and lateral patellar ligaments.

As the stifle joint extends and flexes, the patella glides up and down a groove at the lower end of the femur. This groove is called the trochlea. The trochlea has a prominent medial ridge with a knob-like projection on the upper edge. On the medial side of the patella is a cartilage extension which overlies the medial ridge of the trochlea.

This arrangement allows the stifle to be locked in an extended position. The joint is extended by contraction of the powerful quadriceps femoris muscle, which passes along the front and both sides of the femur to attach to the patella. As the joint is fully extended, the patella glides to the upper limit of the trochlear groove. If the patella is then twisted medially, the knob of the medial ridge of the trochlea projects between the medial and middle patellar ligaments.

This locking mechanism allows the horse to stand for long periods of time without experiencing muscle fatigue. The opposite hind leg is rested.

To unlock the stifle, the horse's weight is shifted to the opposite hind limb. The quadriceps muscle pulls the patella in an upward

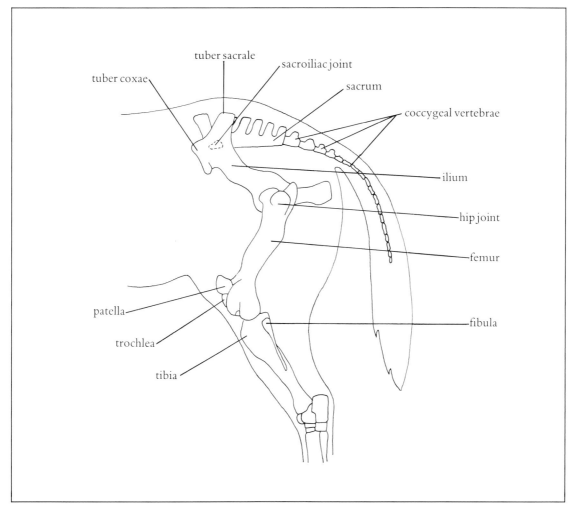

Figure 5.10 *Lateral view of the stifle, hip and sacroiliac joints of the horse*

direction. The patella is then twisted laterally and returned to the trochlear groove.

Intermittent Upward Fixation of the Patella

This is a condition where the horse or pony is temporarily unable to unlock the stifle from the extended position. It can lock for a few strides or for hours at a time. The problem may be experienced in one or both hind limbs.

Young, unfit or poorly muscled animals are particularly susceptible. The condition is common in Shetland ponies and may be hereditary.

Clinical signs

- The stifle and hock cannot be flexed. The horse hops forward with its leg stuck out behind it
- The toe may be dragged along the ground
- In less severe cases, the patella does not lock, but 'catches' with every stride. This is most easily observed when the horse is:
  - lunged at walk with the affected limb on the inside
  - rocked from side to side while standing square
  - walked up and down a hill
- The horse is not usually lame. However, in severe or long-standing cases, the stifle

joint becomes inflamed; lameness and degenerative joint disease may develop.

Treatment

Immediate action

The stifle often unlocks spontaneously after a few strides. If not, the situation can usually be resolved by making the horse jump forwards smartly or by walking it backwards.

Longer-term management

- Improvement of muscle tone. The quadriceps muscle should be strengthened by increasing the amount of exercise and improving the diet of animals in poor condition. Stabled horses and ponies often improve if they are turned out. Where this regime fails, or if the stifle of young, unbroken animals repeatedly locks, surgery may be necessary.
- Corrective surgery. The condition can be corrected by a simple operation, called a medial patellar desmotomy. The medial patellar ligament is cut under local anaesthesia with the horse standing under sedation.

  This technique is now used only as a last resort following reports of complications that can lead to permanent lameness.

Prognosis

The prognosis is favourable when the condition resolves as the horse becomes fitter.

6 Synovial Effusions

Synovial Effusions

Synovial membranes sometimes produce an abnormal amount of synovial fluid in response to low-grade trauma. This can cause a swelling without any heat or lameness.

The examples considered here include:
- joints, e.g. bog spavin, articular windgalls
- tendon sheaths, e.g. tendinous windgalls, thoroughpin
- bursae, e.g. hygroma of the knee, capped hock, capped elbow.

Joints

Bog spavin

Bog spavin is the name given to a synovial effusion of the tibiotarsal joint of the hock. The joint capsule can become markedly distended. One or both hocks may be affected (*Figure 6.1*).

The condition tends to occur in horses with poor hock conformation, e.g. cow hocks, sickle hocks and straight hocks.

Clinical signs

Two fluid-filled swellings develop below the point of the hock:
- the largest is on the front of the hock towards the inside
- the second, smaller swelling is slightly higher up on the outside of the joint.

As these are distensions of the same joint, if one is pressed, the other enlarges. There is no pain or lameness.

Diagnosis

Diagnosis is made on the clinical signs.

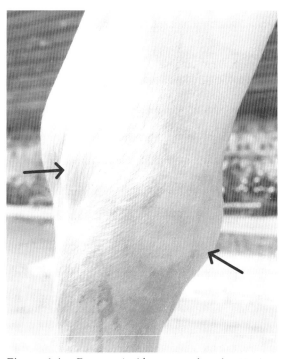

Figure 6.1 *Bog spavin (the arrows show location)*

N.B. Bog spavin must be differentiated from:

- hock sprains
- bone spavin
- osteochondritis dissecans (a developmental abnormality of cartilage and bone in fast-growing horses).

Each of these conditions can also cause enlargement of the tibiotarsal joint. However, they are usually accompanied by lameness, inflammation or radiographic changes.

Treatment

No treatment is necessary. The fluid may be spontaneously resorbed over a period of time. Topical applications, e.g. DMSO and flumethasone may speed up the process.

Draining the swellings is not recommended as it involves invasion of the joint. If they are drained, the swellings often reform, especially where poor conformation is a contributory factor.

Articular windgalls

Articular windgalls (*Figure 6.2*) are distensions of the fetlock joint capsule.

Clinical signs

These swellings can be seen on either side of the limb, between the back of the cannon bone and the suspensory ligament. Pressing the swelling on one side of the joint causes the swelling on the opposite side to enlarge.

They often fluctuate in size according to the exercise programme. In some horses they are only present after a spell of heavy work, whereas in others they are permanent.

Causes

The cause is low-grade trauma of the fetlock joint. Articular windgalls frequently develop

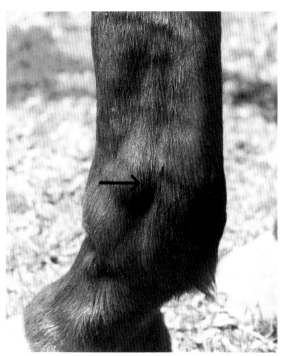

Figure 6.2   *Articular windgall (the arrow shows location)*

in stocky animals with upright conformation. They are also common in horses that work hard.

Treatment

This condition is not usually associated with lameness, and no treatment is necessary.

Where the swelling of the fetlock joint capsule is accompanied by heat and/or lameness, the condition should be fully investigated. The appropriate treatment can then be given.

Tendon Sheaths

Tendon sheaths are long thin sacs of synovial

fluid that surround and protect tendons as they pass over bony prominences.

If production of synovial fluid is increased, the tendon sheath becomes distended. Examples include tendinous windgalls and thoroughpin.

Tendinous windgalls

These are enlargements of the flexor tendon sheath. The swellings occur just above the fetlock, between the suspensory ligament and the flexor tendons (*Figure 6.3*). They are usually larger on the hind limbs.

As with articular windgalls they are not associated with lameness and do not require any treatment.

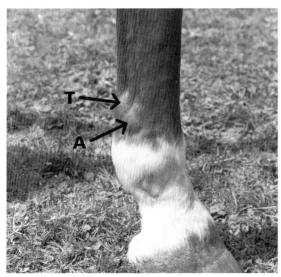

Figure 6.3   *Articular and tendinous windgalls (the arrows show location)*

Thoroughpin

A thoroughpin is a swelling of the tarsal sheath which encloses the deep digital flexor tendon as it passes over the hock. The swelling occurs in front of the Achilles tendon just above the point of the hock (*Figure 6.4*).

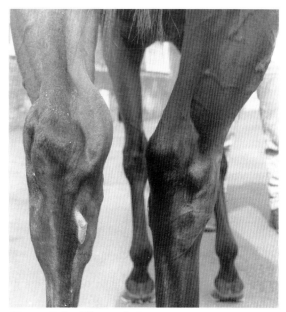

Figure 6.4   *Thoroughpin*

Thoroughpin is often associated with straight hocks.

The swelling may be resorbed over a period of time. Treatment is not necessary, although topical applications, e.g. DMSO and flumethasone are sometimes used to help reduce the swelling.

Bursae

A bursa is a small sac of synovial fluid. Bursae may be congenital or acquired.

Congenital bursae are present in all horses from birth. They are situated where a tendon passes over a bony prominence. The fluid-filled sac cushions the tendon and protects it from the effects of friction.

Acquired bursae are not present in every animal. They develop under the skin as a reaction to repeated trauma. These swellings are usually cold and painless.

The following sections give examples of acquired bursae.

Hygroma of the knee

This is a swelling on the front of the knee.

Causes

These include:
- inadequate bedding
- knocking a fence
- banging the stable door.

Prevention

- Provide a thick, comfortable bed.
- Pad the door with thick foam rubber or replace it with a wooden bar or chain during the day.
- Protect the knee when travelling.

Capped hock

A swelling develops on the point of the hock (*Figure 6.5*).

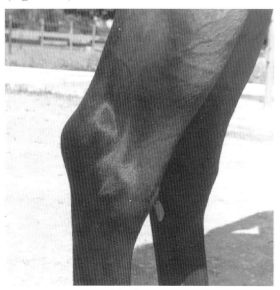

Figure 6.5   *Capped hock*

Causes

A capped hock can be caused by:
- inadequate bedding
- leaning against the stable wall or trailer ramp
- a blow to the point of hock.

Prevention

- Provide a thick, banked bed.
- Protect the hocks when travelling.

Capped elbow

A subcutaneous bursa develops on the elbow.

Causes

It is caused by repeated knocks from the heel of the front shoe when the horse lies down (*Figure 6.6*) or during fast work.

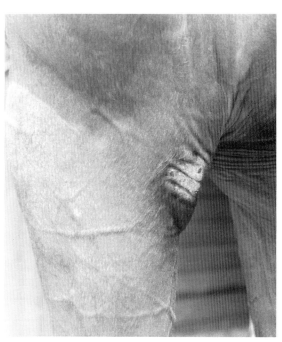

Figure 6.6   *Elbow injury caused by the heels of the front shoes when the horse lies down*

Prevention

Use a sausage boot (*Figure 6.7*) around the pastern.

Treatment of acquired bursae

Removal of the cause

Where the swelling is recognised in the early stages and the cause is removed, no further treatment is necessary.

Topical applications

DMSO and flumethasone, for example, may assist reduction of the swelling.

Drainage

If the swelling is large and unsightly, the fluid can be drained by the vet. The improvement may only be slight or temporary as the swelling often reforms. Effective bandaging of these sites is very difficult.

Surgical removal

Very large swellings that do not respond to treatment and preventive measures can be removed surgically.

Bursitis

Bursitis is inflammation of a bursa. It develops as a sequel to trauma or infection.

Septic bursitis

Examples include:
- fistulous withers, which causes a swelling over the withers that eventually bursts
- infection of a navicular bursa following penetration by a nail. Symptoms include severe lameness and swelling of the lower limb.

Treatment

Drainage must be established together with surgical removal of all dead and infected tissue. Even following radical surgery and intensive antibiotic therapy, the prognosis in both cases is extremely guarded.

Traumatic bursitis

When a bursa is subjected to a hard blow, it may become acutely inflamed.

Symptoms include heat, swelling and a variable degree of lameness. For example, the

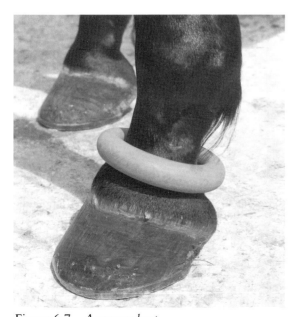

Figure 6.7   *A sausage boot*

bursa which lies close to the fetlock underneath the common digital extensor tendon is often knocked by National Hunt horses.

Treatment

Treatments include:

- rest
- cold therapy
- support bandaging
- anti-inflammatory drugs.

When the inflammation has subsided, the bursa may remain permanently enlarged.

7 Tendon and Ligament Injuries

Structure and Function of Tendons

Tendons are bands of dense white fibrous tissue that connect muscles to bones (*Figure 7.1*). They are made up of parallel bundles of longitudinally aligned collagen fibrils. They have great tensile strength, but are relatively inelastic.

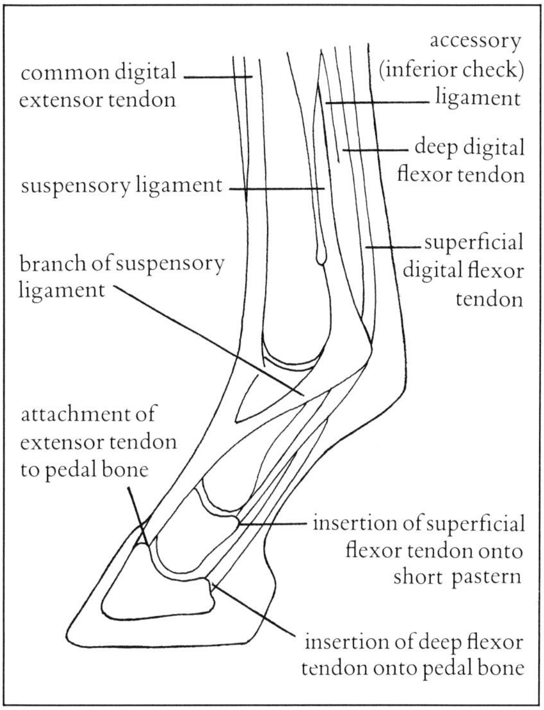

Strains

Strains occur when the tendon is over-stretched. The resultant haemorrhage and inflammation disrupts the normal alignment of the collagen fibrils.

Healing

During the healing process, cells called fibroblasts migrate into the area and produce new collagen. The tendon becomes thickened and bowed (*Figure 7.2*).

The repair collagen (type 3) is not as strong as the original (type 1) collagen and the new fibrils tend to be laid down in a random fashion. The tendon never regains its former strength and is therefore prone to reinjury.

The healing process continues for up to 15 months after the injury occurs.

Figure 7.1   *Tendons and ligaments of the forelimb*

Labels: common digital extensor tendon; suspensory ligament; branch of suspensory ligament; attachment of extensor tendon to pedal bone; accessory (inferior check) ligament; deep digital flexor tendon; superficial digital flexor tendon; insertion of superficial flexor tendon onto short pastern; insertion of deep flexor tendon onto pedal bone

Strains of the Superficial and Deep Digital Flexor Tendons

The narrowest point of the superficial digital

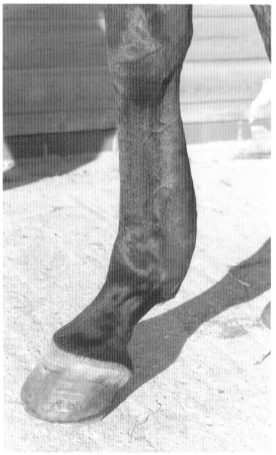

Figure 7.2 *Bowed tendon: severe strain of the superficial digital flexor tendon*

flexor tendon is at the mid-cannon level; this is the commonest site of injury. Strains of this tendon are relatively common in the forelimbs of horses that gallop or jump at speed on variable going, e.g. racehorses, eventers and hunters.

Strains of the deep digital flexor tendon are far less common.

Causes

Predisposing factors which put extra strain on the tendons include:

- *poor conformation*, e.g. long sloping pasterns, overlong toes and 'back at the knee' conformation
- *fatigue* which causes inefficient muscle action and may result in uncoordinated movements
- *working at speed* on hard, uneven ground or in deep mud.

Clinical signs

These vary according to the severity of the strain.

Severe strains

The horse is very lame and the tendon is obviously hot and swollen. It is very painful and even gentle squeezing causes the horse to withdraw the limb.

In the acute stages, the horse may bear very little weight on the affected limb, tending to stand with the knee flexed and the heel slightly raised from the ground.

Where major disruption of the tendon has occurred, the fetlock sinks closer to the ground than normal.

Mild strains

It is possible for a horse to have a moderate degree of tendon damage without being lame.

In these cases, it is *absolutely essential* that the injury is recognised and treated before further damage occurs.

Warning signs include increased warmth and very slight swelling of the tendon.

Diagnosis

Diagnosis is made on the clinical signs. An

ultrasound scanner can be used to determine the extent and severity of the damage.

Treatment

The aims of treatment are to:
- relieve the pain
- reduce the swelling and inflammation
- provide support
- encourage longitudinal alignment of the collagen fibrils.

The treatment programme

The treatment programme begins with box rest and:
- cold therapy
- non-steroidal anti-inflammatory drugs, e.g. phenylbutazone
- support bandaging of both limbs.

This is followed by a long period of rest in the field.

Box rest

The period of box rest is usually 6–8 weeks. The horse *must not* be turned out at this stage as uncontrolled exercise delays healing and will cause further injury.

Controlled exercise

During the period of box rest, short periods of in-hand walking exercise are introduced as soon as the acute inflammation has subsided. This encourages longitudinal alignment of fibroblasts and collagen fibrils and helps prevent adhesions forming between the tendon and the surrounding tissues. The walking is built up to 30 minutes twice daily.

At the end of the eight week period, your vet will re-examine the horse's leg. If it is cool and healing is progressing well, the horse may be turned out or remain stabled and begin light exercise under saddle. The recommended course of action will depend upon the following:
- severity of the injury
- the progress already made
- temperament of the horse
- experience of the rider
- facilities available
- the state of the ground.

For example, where the ground is too hard or muddy for turning out, a 2–3 month extension of the period of box rest with controlled exercise may be beneficial.

Long rest at grass

The horse is then turned away for at least a year. Progress can be monitored using an ultrasound scanner.

Additional treatments

Tendon healing is a slow process and owners and trainers are anxious to resume training at the earliest possible date. A number of other treatments are therefore used to assist the natural healing process. They include:
- physiotherapy, e.g. laser treatment, ultrasound, magnetic field therapy
- injection of irritant substances into the tendon
- tendon splitting
- carbon fibre implants.

Physiotherapy assists with the reduction of soft tissue swelling. However, there is no scientific evidence that any of the other procedures accelerate or improve tendon healing when compared with that achieved by rest, support and controlled exercise.

Prognosis

The prognosis depends on the severity of the initial injury.

Early recognition and treatment of mild strains usually results in the horse being able to resume its former activities.

Horses with more severe tendon damage often recover sufficiently to undertake light work. There is less chance of the tendon standing up to the stresses of racing or three-day eventing.

Strains of the deep digital flexor tendon usually have a more guarded prognosis than strains of the superficial digital flexor tendon.

Bruised Tendons

The flexor tendons are covered only by skin so they are very vulnerable to bruising from kicks or overreaches.

Treatment

The treatment is similar to that described for tendon strains. Where the overlying skin is broken and infection is a complicating factor, antibiotics are administered.

Prognosis

In general, the recovery period is shorter and the prognosis more favourable than for strained tendons.

Prevention

Boots and bandages provide considerable protection, especially when jumping.

Structure and Function of Ligaments

Ligaments are bands of tough, fibrous tissue that support the joints and hold the bones in place.

Injuries to these structures should be treated promptly to minimise the risk of permanent damage.

Sprain of the Suspensory Ligament

The suspensory ligament (*Figure 7.3*) supports the fetlock joint.

In the forelimb its origin is the lower row of knee bones and the top of the cannon bone. It runs down the back of the cannon bone as a flat band and then divides into lateral and

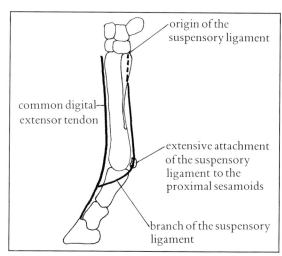

Figure 7.3   *Position of the suspensory ligament*

medial branches. Each branch attaches to one of the proximal sesamoids before running obliquely across the long pastern to join the common digital extensor tendon.

The suspensory ligament can be seen and palpated just behind the cannon and splint bones on either side of the limb.

Suspensory problems often occur in association with splint bone and sesamoid injuries because of the close proximity to these structures.

Sprains are incurred during fast work and are commonly seen in the forelimbs of hunters and eventers. The usual site of injury is close to the fetlock where the ligament divides.

Clinical signs

- Lameness.
- Heat.
- Soft tissue swelling.
- Thickening of the ligament.
- Pain on palpation.

The ligament can also become inflamed close to its origin on the cannon bone. In these cases the signs are less obvious but should still be regarded as serious. There is often little or no swelling and lameness may only be apparent after hard work.

Diagnosis

Diagnosis of suspensory sprains is made on the clinical signs. An ultrasound scanner can be used to show the extent and severity of the damage.

In cases where the pain arises from the origin of the suspensory ligament, diagnosis is made by infiltration of local anaesthetic around the region, whereupon the horse becomes sound.

In severe cases, new bone is formed and can be seen on radiographs.

Treatment

The aims are to:
- relieve pain
- reduce inflammation and swelling
- provide support
- allow sufficient time for healing.

This is achieved by:
- box rest
- cold treatment for the first 48 hours
- support bandaging
- administration of non-steroidal anti-inflammatory drugs, e.g. phenylbutazone
- ultrasound or laser treatment.

The period of box rest is usually 6–8 weeks. As the acute inflammation subsides, the horse can be walked out in hand. This helps to prevent adhesions and should be gradually increased to 30 minutes twice daily.

At the end of the period of box rest, the horse must be re-examined by the vet. Provided the leg is cool and healing is progressing satisfactorily, the horse is turned away for at least six months.

Prognosis

A suspensory sprain is a serious injury. The prognosis depends on the severity of the damage and the use of the horse. With adequate rest, many horses are able to return to their former work.

Sprain of the Accessory Ligament of the Deep Ditigal Flexor Tendon

Sprains of the deep digital flexor tendon are

uncommon. The accessory (inferior check) ligament, however, is subject to sprains.

Anatomy

This ligament lies between the suspensory ligament and the deep digital flexor tendon. It runs from the carpal ligament at the back of the knee to join the deep digital flexor tendon halfway down the cannon bone.

Clinical signs

These include:
- slight to moderate lameness
- heat over the area
- swelling and eventual thickening of the ligament

Diagnosis

Diagnosis is made on the clinical signs.
    The extent and severity of the injury is determined using an ultrasound scanner.

Treatment

A sprain of the accessory ligament should be treated as a serious injury, even though the lameness may only be slight.
    Treatment is as described for a tendon sprain, but recovery is normally complete within 3–6 months.

Prognosis

With early diagnosis and treatment the prognosis is good.

Curb

A curb (*Figure 7.4*) is a swelling that develops at the back of the hock when the plantar ligament is sprained.
    This ligament attaches to the calcaneus, the fourth tarsal bone and the top of the lateral splint bone (*Figure 7.5*).

Causes and predisposing factors

- *Poor hock conformation*, e.g. cow hocks and sickle hocks, predisposes a horse to developing curbs by putting additional strain on the plantar ligament.
- *Strenuous exercise* including bucking and kicking.

Clinical signs

In the acute stages there may be:
- heat
- swelling
- mild lameness which increases with exercise
- a tendency to stand with the heel slightly raised.

However, many horses that develop curbs do not become lame.

Treatment

Treatment may include:
- rest
- cold therapy in the early stages
- non-steroidal anti-inflammatory drugs, e.g. phenylbutazone
- topical applications, e.g. DMSO and flumethasone, to reduce the swelling.

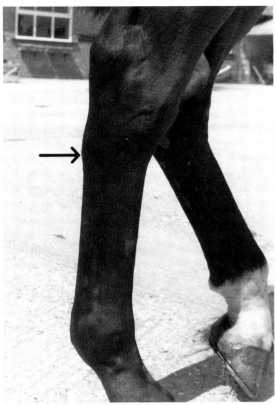

Figure 7.4 *A curb (the arrow shows location)*

Prognosis

The prognosis is good unless the hock conformation is so poor that the ligament suffers recurrent sprains.

The swelling is usually permanent due to thickening of the ligament by fibrous tissue. In severe cases new bone is formed.

N.B. Some horses have a very prominent proximal (top) end to the lateral splint bone. This is known as a false curb. It can be differentiated from true curbs by close examination or x-rays.

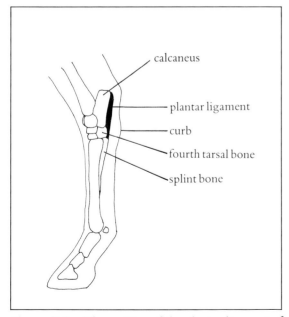

Figure 7.5 *The position of the plantar ligament of the hock*

8 Bone Injuries

Periostitis

Periostitis is inflammation of the periosteum which is the thin membrane that covers bone.

The periosteum is composed of two layers:
- an outer fibrous layer
- an inner cellular layer containing blood vessels and cells that can differentiate into *osteoblasts*. These cells are able to produce new bone.

The periosteum is important for:
- attachment of tendons and ligaments to bone
- nutrition of bone
- growth of young bone
- repair of bone fractures.

Causes

The periosteum can become inflamed following a direct blow or tearing of the attached ligaments.

The resultant haemorrhage lifts the periosteum away from the bone and this stimulates the osteoblasts to produce new bone.

Clinical signs

A tender, bony swelling develops. This is often accompanied by heat and inflammation of the surrounding soft tissue.

As the inflammation subsides, the bony lump remodels, becoming smaller and painless.

Radiographic changes

The new bone is visible from approximately two weeks after the injury occurs. Where the outline appears fuzzy, the inflammation is still active. Once it has settled, the new bone acquires a smooth contour.

Examples of periostitis include sore shins and splints.

Sore (bucked) Shins

In this condition the front of the cannon bone becomes inflamed and sore (*Figure 8.1*). The disease is characteristically seen in two- and three-year-old Thoroughbreds.

Causes

It occurs when immature bones are subjected to the stresses of training.

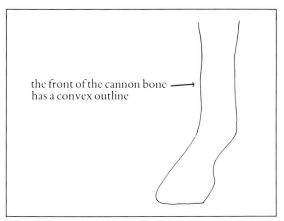

Figure 8.1   *Sore shin*

Microfractures and haemorrhage develop under the periosteum at the front of the cannon bone.

Clinical signs

- Heat.
- Pain when pressure is applied.
- A convex outline to the front of the cannon bone.
- An alteration of gait, ranging from a slight shortening of stride to obvious lameness. This becomes more apparent after work.

Diagnosis

Diagnosis is made on the clinical signs.

Treatment

Treatment may include:
- box rest, with short periods of in-hand walking exercise on soft ground
- cold therapy in the early stages
- non-steroidal anti-inflammatory drugs to reduce the inflammation and pain
- magnetic field therapy.

Prognosis

With correct treatment, the prognosis is good, although recovery may take up to three months.

After the inflammation has subsided, the outline of the bone may remain convex.

Splints

A splint is a bony enlargement of a splint bone. Each limb has a splint bone attached to either side of the cannon bone by a strong, interosseus ligament (*Figure 8.2*).

In a young horse, this ligament is subject to strains and tears, which result in bleeding and proliferation of fibrous tissue. The periosteum of the splint bone becomes inflamed and new bone is produced.

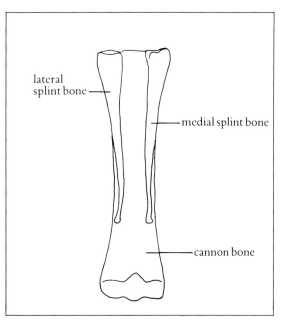

Figure 8.2   *Back view of the left cannon bone and splint bones of a horse*

Causes

Any of the following factors can contribute to the development of splints:
- working on hard ground
- a direct blow to the splint bone, e.g. interference from the opposite limb or a kick from another horse
- poor conformation
- faulty trimming and shoeing.

Clinical signs

Splints most commonly occur on the medial side (inside) of the forelimb, approximately 7.5 cm below the knee.

There is heat, swelling and pain over the splint bone. Pressing the site causes pain.

Horses developing a splint show variable degrees of lameness. They may be:
- sound
- sound at walk, lame at trot
- lame at walk and trot.

Lameness from developing splints tends to increase with work, especially over hard or rough ground.

As the splint settles down, the swelling becomes smaller but harder and the lameness resolves.

Complications

- New bone formed high up on the splint bone may affect the knee joint.
- New bone can interfere with the suspensory ligament and cause lameness.

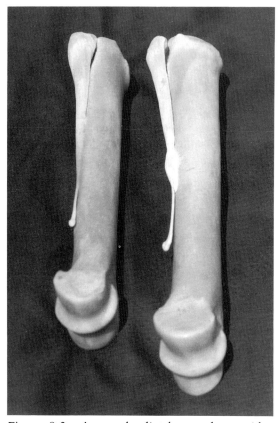

Figure 8.3 *A normal splint bone and one with a 'splint'*

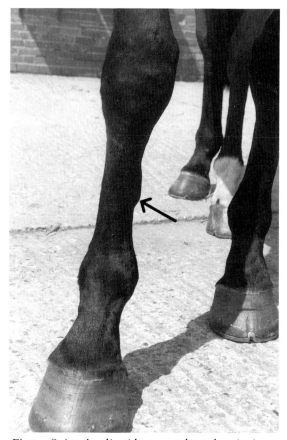

Figure 8.4 *A splint (the arrow shows location)*

Diagnosis

Diagnosis is made on the clinical signs and confirmed by radiography.

Radiographs are useful because they:

- show whether the splint is active
- determine the extent of new bone growth and its position in relation to the suspensory ligament and knee joint
- reduce the chance of a fracture being overlooked.

Treatment

Cold treatment and support bandaging

These are beneficial in the early stages.

Non-steroidal anti-inflammatory drugs

These drugs, e.g. phenylbutazone help reduce the inflammation.

Box rest

Box rest is advised. Uncontrolled field exercise will increase the inflammation and hence the risk of complications. The period of box rest is variable; each case must be individually assessed.

Topical applications

Applications such as DMSO and flumethasone may be applied two or three times daily when the cold treatment is finished.

Surgery

There are three indications for surgical removal of the bony swelling:

- if the splint interferes with the suspensory ligament
- if it encroaches on the knee joint
- if it is so large that it is repeatedly knocked by the opposite limb.

Surgery is *not* recommended for cosmetic reasons alone as the trauma associated with splint removal occasionally causes even larger bony lumps to form.

Return to work

Once the condition has resolved, the horse can be brought back slowly into full work. The use of brushing boots or exercise bandages is recommended and working on hard ground should be avoided.

Prevention

- Avoid working young horses on hard ground.
- Use brushing boots for lungeing and schooling, especially if the horse moves close in front.
- Make sure the feet are correctly trimmed and shod on a regular basis.

By the time a horse is six years old, the ligament is much more stable. It is gradually strengthened by deposition of bone within its substance.

Carpitis

Carpitis is inflammation of the knee (*Figure 8.5*).

The bones, the joint capsule or the ligaments may be affected, and the condition can progress to degenerative joint disease.

Causes

The disease may be caused by:
- acute injury, e.g. a fall or knocking a fence
- working young animals with immature bones, e.g. two- and three-year-old race-horses
- poor knee conformation which puts abnormal strains on the joints and ligaments.

Clinical signs

These include some of the following:
- lameness
- shortening of the stride
- a base-wide gait when the condition affects both knees
- distension of the joint capsule
- bony enlargement of the front of the knee (*Figure 8.6*)
- pain when firm pressure is applied
- severe pain on flexion (the horse may rear to evade the pain)
- reduced degree of flexion
- a tendency to stand with the knee slightly flexed.

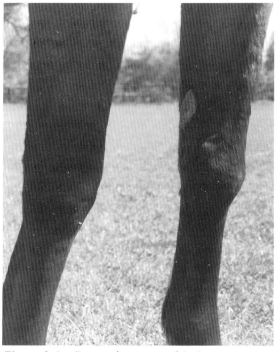

Figure 8.6   *Bony enlargement of the knee*

Diagnosis

Diagnosis is made on:
- clinical signs
- intra-articular nerve blocks

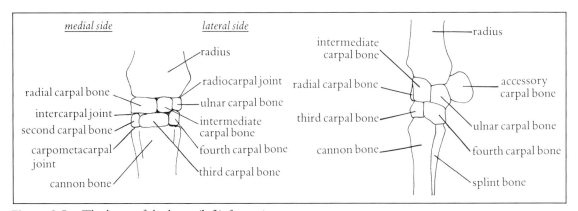

Figure 8.5   *The bones of the knee:* (left) *front view* (right) *lateral view*

- synovial fluid analysis
- radiography (*Figure 8.7*)

It is possible for the joint surfaces to remain normal despite extensive new bone growth on the front of the knee.

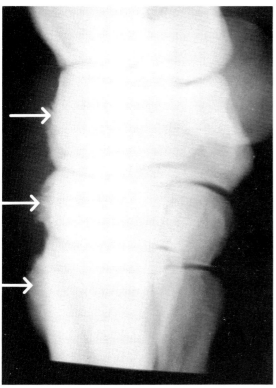

Figure 8.7 *Carpitis: radiograph showing extensive new bone growth on the front of the knee (the arrows show location)*

Treatment

Treatment may include:
- box rest with short periods of in-hand walking exercise
- cold treatment in the early stages
- non-steroidal anti-inflammatory drugs, e.g. phenylbutazone to reduce pain and inflammation
- ultrasound, laser or magnetic field therapy
- topical applications of, for example, DMSO and flumethasone
- flexing the knee several times each day to keep the joint mobile and prevent adhe-

sions forming
- if early degenerative joint disease is suspected, the joint may be injected with sodium hyaluronate or polysulphated glycosaminoglycan.

Stable management

A thick bed should be provided to minimise the risk of further trauma when lying down.

Prognosis

The prognosis is reasonably good if the condition was caused by a direct blow to the knee and there is no joint involvement.

If the cause of the disease cannot be removed, e.g. conformation faults, the prognosis is more guarded.

Sesamoiditis

Sesamoiditis is inflammation of the sesamoid bones.

Anatomy

There are two proximal sesamoid bones at the back of the fetlock, one on either side of the limb.

The upper edge of each bone is firmly attached to the medial or lateral branch of the suspensory ligament and the lower edge is attached to the long and short pastern by a number of ligaments.

The two sesamoid bones are joined by the intersesamoidean ligament.

Causes

Sesamoiditis is usually caused by:
- tearing of the suspensory or distal ligament attachments when the fetlock joint is over-extended. This occurs when tired horses gallop or jump at speed. Overlong toes increase susceptibility to the injury
- direct trauma, e.g. an overreach.

In either case, the sesamoid bones can fracture.

Clinical signs

The degree of lameness depends on the severity of the injury.
- It is worse on hard ground and at the onset of exercise.
- The horse tends to move in an upright fashion as extension of the fetlock pulls the damaged ligaments and is painful.
- Flexion of the fetlock may be painful and increase the degree of lameness.
- There is heat and soft tissue swelling at the back of the fetlock.
- The horse is sensitive to firm pressure over the area.
- As the soft tissue swelling subsides, the suspensory ligament may remain permanently thickened close to its sesamoid attachment, altering the outline of the fetlock joint.

X-ray findings include:
- new bone laid down on the sesamoid bones or in the branches of the suspensory ligament
- changes in bone density
- increased number of vascular channels in the bone.

With the exception of a fracture, these x-ray changes will not be visible until at least three weeks after the injury has occurred.

Treatment

- In the acute stages, cold treatment and support bandaging are beneficial.
- Anti-inflammatory drugs, e.g. phenylbutazone, help to reduce the swelling.
- Box rest is usually recommended for a period of up to six weeks.
- A programme of corrective trimming should be started for horses with poor hoof conformation.
- The horse should then be turned away for several months.

Prognosis

The prognosis depends on the severity of the injury. It is usually guarded as the condition tends to recur.

Fractures

A fracture can be defined as a break in the continuity of a bone (*Figure 8.8*).

Recent advances in surgical techniques, repair materials, and anaesthesia mean that a wide range of fractures can now be treated.

The prognosis depends on which bone is involved and the nature of the fracture.

Splint Bone Fracture

Fracture of a splint bone (*Figure 8.9*) is a

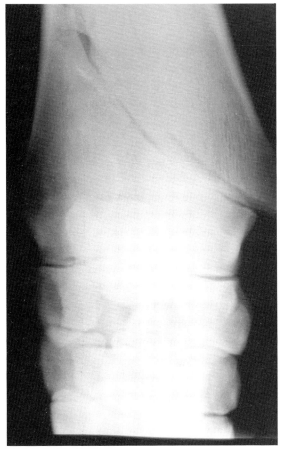

Figure 8.8   *Fracture of the radius*

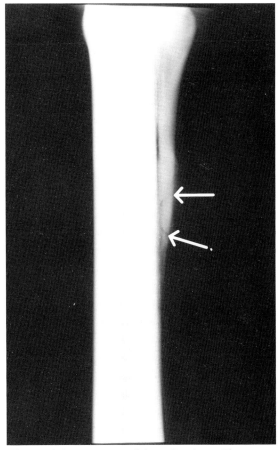

Figure 8.9   *Fracture of the splint bone (the arrows show location)*

relatively common injury. The fracture usually occurs in the lower third of the bone.

Causes

These include:
- being struck by the foot of the opposite limb
- a kick from another horse
- a penetrating wound.

Clinical signs

The symptoms are similar to those shown by a horse developing splints, i.e.:
- heat, swelling and pain over the splint bone
- pain when the fracture site is pressed
- a variable degree of lameness.

Diagnosis

Diagnosis is made on the clinical signs and confirmed by radiography.

Complications

- Infection may enter an open wound and

become established in the bone (osteomyelitis).

- A small fragment may separate from the splint bone, lose its blood supply and die. In these cases, pus discharges onto the skin surface through a sinus which will not heal until the piece of bone is removed.

A support bandage is necessary to prevent further trauma.

Other fractures are generally treated by surgical removal of the distal (lower) fragment and any bone chips. When infection is present, antibiotics are administered prior to surgery.

Treatment

This depends on the nature of the fracture and the presence of any complicating factors.

A simple fracture with no overlying skin wound usually heals with six weeks box rest.

Prognosis

The prognosis is good unless new bone interferes with the knee joint or the suspensory ligament.

9 The Horse's Back

Back Pain

Back pain may originate from the vertebrae, the ligaments, the muscles or the skin.

Causes and predisposing factors

Certain types of conformation predispose a horse to back pain. Animals with long backs are susceptible to muscle and ligament strains; those with short backs are more prone to vertebral problems.

The common causes of back pain include:
- falls, jumping awkwardly, slipping
- incorrectly fitted or poorly maintained saddles
- pain elsewhere in the body causing the horse to alter its gait and put unusual stresses on the back muscles
- bad riding.

Clinical signs

Behavioural changes include:
- resentment of grooming and saddling. The horse may kick out or attempt to lie down as the girth is tightened
- dipping or arching of the back when mounted
- loss of enthusiasm for work
- general stiffness, especially when turning or working on a circle
- reluctance to stay on the bit
- poor hind limb impulsion and failure to track up
- swishing of the tail or carrying it to one side
- refusal to jump or poor jumping technique
- bucking when the rider's leg is applied
- reluctance to rein back.

Back pain may cause intermittent, bilateral hind limb lameness. It rarely causes lameness in one hind limb.

Diagnosis

In some cases, finding the painful area and pinpointing the cause is relatively straightforward. In other cases, reaching a specific diagnosis is extremely difficult. This is because:
- the symptoms often occur intermittently and could also apply to a number of other conditions
- owing to the depth of the muscles and ligaments, it is not always possible to locate the tender spot by palpation of the back.

How to examine a horse's back

The horse can be examined for back pain using the following tests.

1) View the back from both sides to see if there is any localised muscle swelling or wasting.

2) Stand the horse square and view it from behind, standing on a milk crate if necessary.

   Check that the spine is not curved to one side. Lateral curvature is indicative of vertebral injury or muscle spasm.

3) Now feel the muscles on either side of the spine from the withers to the tail. Begin by gently stroking your hand along the back so the horse stays relaxed. Then run the flat of your fingers over the muscles either side of the spine, two or three times, gradually increasing the pressure. Firm pressure on a painful spot usually provokes a reaction from the horse. The muscle may go into spasm and feel much harder than the adjacent muscle. If the pain is severe, the horse will put its ears back and try to move away. Alternatively, it may grunt and dip its back or even lash out.

4) Flexion of the spine is tested in two ways:

   a) Run a ballpoint pen along either side of the spine from the withers to the tail. On reaching the loins, the horse will dip its back. As you pass over the highest point of the quarters, the horse humps its back. These reactions are completely normal.

      If the horse experiences pain, it may tense its muscles and hold its back rigid or demonstrate its discomfort in some other obvious way. Some placid, thick-skinned horses and ponies show no response to this test; this should not be interpreted as a sign that something is wrong.

   b) To test lateral flexion of the spine, run a ballpoint pen down from the middle of the back, over the top of the ribcage. The horse will normally curve its spine away from you.

5) Back the horse in a straight line for four or five steps. Animals with back pain often show resistance.

6) Finally, turn the horse in a very tight circle on both reins and see if it can cross one hind leg in front of the other.

Interpretation

Interpretation of the horse's response to these tests is not always straightforward.

Horses with previous back injuries may associate the examination procedure with discomfort and become tense and uncooperative. Thin-skinned horses often show very exaggerated responses which give a false impression of back pain.

If you are uncertain, or find any evidence of back pain, the horse should be examined by the vet.

Cold Backs

The term 'cold-backed' is used to describe horses that persistently dip their backs and hindquarters when mounted. They often stagger or move stiffly for a couple of strides and then work normally.

Causes

This reaction may be a sign of discomfort or it may simply be a habit.

Action

In order to be sure that nothing serious is wrong, a veterinary examination is essential.

Rest makes no difference to this behaviour but the following steps may help.

1) Ask a saddler to check the fitting and stuffing of the saddle at regular intervals.
2) Use a thick, fleecy numnah or shock absorbing pad under the saddle.
3) Tack the horse up 10 minutes before mounting. Make sure the horse stays warm while waiting to be ridden.
4) Try lungeing the horse gently for five minutes before mounting.
5) Always mount from a mounting block. A heavy rider mounting slowly and awkwardly puts a lot of strain on the horse's muscles and balance.
6) Do not sit heavily in the saddle when you mount. Stand up in the stirrups and ask the horse to walk forwards. Then gently lower your weight onto the saddle after some 20 to 50 metres.
7) Wherever possible, avoid walking downhill immediately after mounting.

These measures also apply to horses recovering from back injuries.

Strained Muscles

Causes

Strains of the back muscles usually result from falls, awkward movements or overexertion.

Clinical signs

These include:
- areas of muscle spasm
- soreness on palpation
- dipping of the back when mounted
- abnormal stiffness of the back and hind-

quarters when lunged or ridden
- reduced hind limb impulsion.

Diagnosis

Diagnosis is made on the clinical signs.
In addition:
- faradism may be used to locate the painful muscle group(s)
- blood tests will show elevated levels of creatine kinase (CK) and aspartate aminotransferase (AST) when the muscle damage is severe.

Treatment

1) Rest

The most important and effective treatment is rest. The recovery time depends on the severity of the injury. Severe strains may require up to 12 weeks off work.

2) Non-steroidal anti-inflammatory drugs

These drugs relieve the pain and inflammation in the acute stages.

3) Manipulation

Manipulation can relieve muscle spasm.

4) Heat treatment, ultrasound and faradism

These assist healing. Your vet will recommend the appropriate programme of physiotherapy.

5) Controlled exercise

During the latter part of the recovery phase, the horse may be lunged to strengthen the muscles before ridden work commences. The demands made on the horse should be increased gradually.

Overriding of the Dorsal Spinous Processes

Each of the thoracic and lumbar vertebrae has a dorsal spinous process (*Figure 9.1*). If the alignment of the vertebrae is altered by an injury or a fall, the spines may touch or overlap each other (*Figure 9.2*).

This condition is most commonly seen in the caudal thoracic (mid-back) region of short-backed horses.

Clinical signs

There may be no clinical signs until a couple of years after the injury. The horse often begins to show signs of back pain as its schooling becomes more advanced and physically demanding.

The symptoms are extremely variable and can be intermittent.

They include:
- resentment of grooming and saddling
- lying down after saddling
- leaping forward when asked to move off after being mounted
- arching the back
- discomfort going downhill
- refusing to jump
- muscle spasm

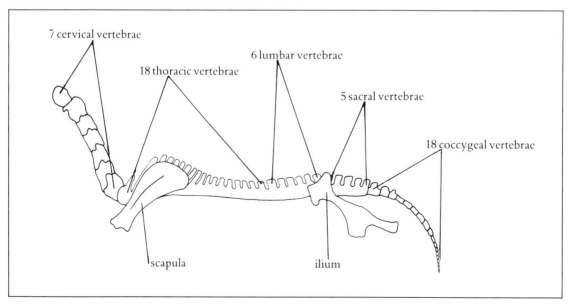

Figure 9.1   *The spine of the horse showing the normal alignment of the dorsal spinous processes*

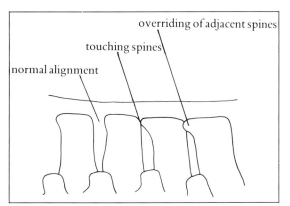

normal alignment

touching spines

overriding of adjacent spines

Figure 9.2 *Impingement and overriding of the dorsal spinous processes*

Some horses show pain when pressure is applied to the back. In other cases the clinical examination reveals nothing abnormal.

Diagnosis

The diagnosis has to be confirmed radiographically and very powerful x-ray equipment is needed.

The x-ray features include:
- less space than normal between adjacent spinous processes
- impingement or overriding of adjacent processes
- remodelling of the affected processes.

Treatment

1) Rest

Some horses improve with six months rest.

2) Non-steroidal anti-inflammatory drugs (e.g. phenylbutazone)

These may relieve the discomfort sufficiently for the horse to continue light work.

3) Surgery

Removal of the tops of one or two dorsal spinous processes results in a return to full activity in some cases.

The surgery is very specialised. There is a risk of complications and no guarantee that the outcome will be successful.

Prognosis

The prognosis is guarded. Affected horses are unable to perform athletically but may be suitable for light hacking.

Saddle Pressure

Pressure from a saddle is a common cause of back pain.

Treatment

Most horses make a full recovery after two weeks without ridden exercise.

A saddler should see the horse to assess the condition and fitting of the saddle.

This subject is covered in more detail later (see Chapter 15).

Sacroiliac Strain

The sacroiliac joint connects the pelvic girdle to the vertebral column (*Figure 5.10*).

All the power from the hind limbs is transmitted to the vertebral column through this joint. It is therefore designed for stability and there is normally no movement between the bones.

Causes and predisposing factors

Horses with long backs and weak hindquarters are prone to sacroiliac strains. The injury is usually the result of slipping or a fall.

Clinical signs

These may include:
- shortening of the hind limb stride and failure to track up
- stiffness
- lack of hind limb impulsion
- intermittent dragging of the toe
- slight to moderate hind limb lameness
- holding the tail to the affected side
- pain when the tuber coxae is pressed because this rotates the pelvis and moves the joint
- asymmetry of the tuber sacrale and the tuber coxae on each side when viewed from behind (*Figure 9.3*)
- movement of one or both of the tuber sacrale when walking
- muscle wasting.

The horse must be made to stand square on a level surface when the symmetry of the pelvis is assessed.

Diagnosis

Diagnosis is made on the clinical signs.
N.B. Many horses with healed sacroiliac

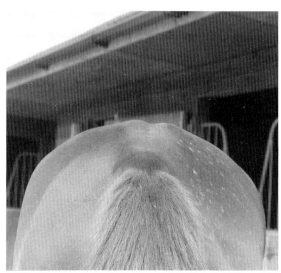

Figure 9.3   *Asymmetry of the tuber sacrale and tuber coxae when viewed from behind*

injuries have slight asymmetry of the bony prominences of the pelvis, but are sound.

Treatment

Treatment begins with six weeks of complete box rest. The horse is then slowly brought back into work. An exercise programme is devised to strengthen the muscles of the hind limbs and the back over a period of time.

Prognosis

The prognosis is guarded after a severe strain as the joint is susceptible to reinjury. Some horses remain slightly unlevel due to instability of the joint, but do not appear to experience any pain.

10 Other Conditions Affecting Movement

Azoturia

Azoturia, or equine rhabdomyolysis, is a condition where certain muscle groups seize up and the horse experiences painful, cramp-like symptoms. The muscles of the loins and quarters are most commonly affected.

It can vary in severity, the horse experiencing symptoms ranging from a slight stiffness of gait to being unable to move at all. In extreme cases, collapse and death occur.

The disease is also referred to as tying-up, set-fast, exertional myopathy, paralytic myoglobinuria, and exertional rhabdomyolysis.

Clinical signs

The symptoms characteristically occur within 10–15 minutes of the start of the exercise.

They include:
- excessive sweating
- hindquarters adopting a rolling action from side to side. If exercise continues, the fetlocks and hocks become flexed so the quarters gradually sink
- a worried expression, with increasing reluctance to move forward
- exaggerated respiration; the horse starts to blow
- increased heart rate
- slight increase in temperature

- pawing the ground and mild colicky signs when allowed to stop
- repeated attempts to urinate, as adopting the normal stance is difficult. Urine varies in colour from normal, through reddish brown to dark chocolate according to the degree of muscle damage
- resentment of pressure on the gluteal and lumbar muscles which may appear swollen and feel hard to touch.

Immediate action

- *Stop* the horse as soon as the gait begins to alter. Forcing the horse to move will only increase the muscle damage.
- Put rugs or coats over the horse's back to keep it warm.
- Arrange transport home in a low-loading trailer.

When to call the vet

Call the vet immediately the condition is suspected.

Diagnosis

Diagnosis is made on clinical signs, the history and laboratory tests.

When muscle cells are damaged, creatine

kinase (CK) and aspartate aminotransferase (AST) leak from the cells into the blood-stream.

The vet will take a blood sample to determine the level of these enzymes which becomes higher as the muscle damage increases.

Causes

The condition is far from fully understood and is still the subject of research and debate.

Carbohydrate overloading

This is the traditional theory. A resting horse on full rations builds up a high concentration of muscle glycogen. When the horse is taken out and commences fast work, a rapid build up of lactic acid damages the muscle fibres. A pigment called myoglobin released from the damaged fibres is responsible for the discoloured urine.

This theory oversimplifies the real situation.

Vitamin and mineral deficiencies

Vitamin E and selenium deficiencies are well known as the cause of muscle problems in other species.

However, there is no proof that a deficiency is responsible for azoturia.

Electrolyte imbalance

The role of calcium, sodium and potassium is currently under investigation as electrolyte imbalance can affect the normal function of nerves and muscles.

Inadequate blood supply

Recent studies indicate that the cause of the condition is inadequate blood supply to the muscle fibres.

It is possible that changes in diet, exercise programmes, climate, stress and a variety of other factors result in altered fluid and electrolyte balance which in turn affects the blood supply to particular muscle groups.

Other theories which have been investigated include:

Hormonal disturbance

There is no evidence that this is a cause.

Temperament

Nervous, excitable horses seem to be particularly at risk.

Genetic factors

A hereditary predisposition has been suggested; there is not enough evidence to support or refute this hypothesis.

Viral infection

Susceptibility in the recovery stages is being investigated.

Treatment

The aim of treatment is to:
- minimise the pain and anxiety
- prevent further muscle damage

- restore fluid and electrolyte balance
- maintain adequate kidney perfusion to minimise myoglobin accumulation in the tubules. Myoglobin is toxic and can cause permanent kidney damage.

The medication and management of affected animals varies with the severity of the condition.

Treatment may include:
- analgesic and anti-inflammatory drugs
- a tranquillizer
- fluid therapy.

Fluid therapy

Electrolyte solutions are added to the drinking water. Fresh water should also be provided.

Recumbent horses require oral and intravenous therapy.

Traditional treatment

This includes vitamin E and selenium; their therapeutic value is now being questioned however.

Care of the patient

In the acute stage of the disease, the horse should be stabled, because even gentle exercise causes further damage to the muscles.

The horse must be kept warm and dry in a well ventilated box that is free from draughts. A thick, dry bed should be provided.

The feed should be reduced to hay, water and, if necessary, horse and pony cubes. Your vet will recommend a diet suited to your horse's needs.

The period of box rest depends on the severity of muscle damage and the rate of recovery. This is monitored by regular blood tests.

Gentle walking exercise in hand is introduced as the horse recovers. Sensible horses may be turned out for a couple of hours providing they are kept warm. Excitable horses should remain stabled as bucking and galloping can cause further muscle damage.

Work should not recommence until the muscle enzymes have returned to normal levels. This is likely to take at least two weeks.

Prevention

Once affected, some horses are susceptible to recurrent attacks of azoturia.

Preventive measures include:

Feed

- Feed a well-balanced diet. Good quality hay, grass and low energy cubes should form the bulk of the ration.
- Rations should be reduced the night before, and on, a day off. Do not increase the feed if an extra strenuous day's work is planned.
- Do not feed large quantities of bran; the high phosphorus content binds with the calcium in the diet, making it unavailable to the horse.
- Avoid sudden changes in diet.
- Specially formulated electrolyte solutions are now commercially available for high-performance horses. When administered prior to stressful situations, e.g. endurance riding or racing, they may help prevent the disease in horses at risk.

Exercise

Fitness training programmes must be carefully planned so that the demands on the horse are increased gradually.

- Do not suddenly increase the speed or duration of exercise.
- Always warm up gently before commencing fast work.
- Try to avoid short bursts of fast exercise.
- Use an exercise sheet to keep the horse warm in wet or cold weather.

Stable management

- Avoid long periods of confinement in the stable.
- Where possible turn the horse out each day and *always* on his day off.

Possible complications

- Muscle wasting will occur in horses suffering from repeated attacks of azoturia. These horses reach a stage where they are unable to work.
- Kidney failure and death occur in severe cases.

Lymphangitis

Lymphangitis is inflammation of the lymph vessels.

The lymphatic system is a network of small vessels that drain excess tissue fluid from all parts of the body. It plays a vital role in removing inflammatory products from injured or infected sites. The fluid is filtered by the lymph nodes (glands) and eventually re-enters the circulation as the lymph vessels join up and drain into a large vein near the heart.

Causes

Infection is usually the cause of the condition. A small scab or old injury can often be found on the lower part of the affected limb. The hind limbs are most commonly involved.

Clinical signs

- Marked swelling of one or more limbs. The swelling usually begins at the pastern and rapidly extends to the elbow or stifle. The upper limit of the swelling may be clearly demarcated as a prominent ridge.

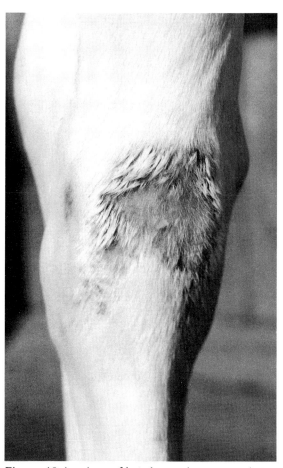

Figure 10.1   *Area of hair loss and serum exudation following an acute attack of lymphangitis. The swelling has subsided*

Over a period of 24 hours, the limb may become 2–3 times its normal size.

- Distended lymph vessels appear very prominent on the inside of the limb. The lymph nodes are enlarged.
- Yellow serum may exude from the skin in several places (*Figure 10.1*).
- The condition is very painful and affected horses move very stiffly. In severe cases little or no weight is placed on the affected limb and the animal is reluctant to move.
- Some horses become very distressed. Additional symptoms may include:
  - sweating
  - trembling
  - blowing
  - loss of appetite
  - a raised body temperature

When to call the vet

Call the vet as soon as the condition is suspected.

Treatment

Prompt, vigorous treatment is required as fibrous tissue builds up with each episode and the leg may become permanently thickened (*Figure 10.2*).

The treatment may include:
- antibiotics to control the infection
- non-steroidal anti-inflammatory drugs (e.g. phenylbutazone) to reduce the soft tissue swelling and relieve the pain
- gentle exercise in hand or at grass to improve circulation and reduce the swelling
- diuretics to increase fluid excretion.

Diet

Feed a low protein diet, e.g. poor grass, mashes and hay.

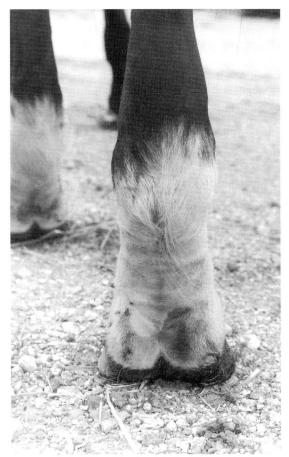

Figure 10.2 *Permanently thickened leg following repeated attacks of lymphangitis*

Prognosis

Once a horse has had lymphangitis the condition may recur.

Pregnant mares

The lymphatic vessels in front of the udder of a pregnant mare sometimes become distended in the late stages of pregnancy. The swelling usually disperses shortly after foaling.

No action is normally required beyond ensuring the mare has plenty of opportunity for exercise. If you are worried or the swelling is causing discomfort, call the vet.

Tetanus

Tetanus is a life-threatening disease caused by the bacterium *Clostridium tetani*. Spores of this bacterium are widespread in the environment and are found in dust, faeces and soil. If they invade a wound which has necrotic (dead) tissue and no oxygen, the bacteria produce a potent toxin. This enters the bloodstream and migrates along peripheral nerves to the central nervous system. It causes muscle spasm and paralysis. The disease is usually fatal.

High risk situations

Injuries which most commonly lead to infection include:
- puncture wounds of the hoof
- stake wounds
- deep thorn penetrations.

The disease is also associated with:
- metritis (uterine infection) following a retained placenta

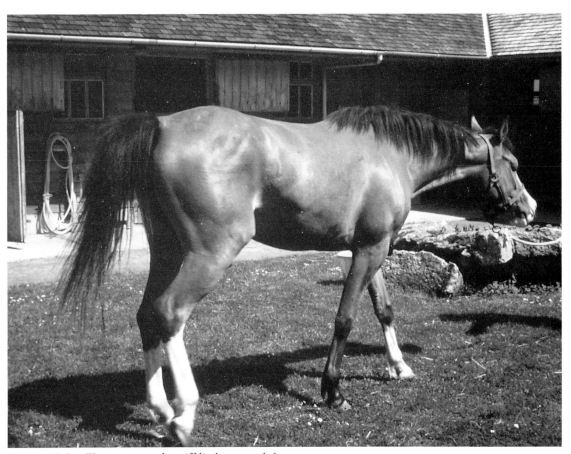

Figure 10.3   *Tetanus: note the stiff limbs, extended neck and raised tail head*

- post-castration infections
- umbilical infections in the foal.

In each case there is an anaerobic environment suitable for bacterial multiplication.

Clinical signs

The incubation period is variable, but clinical signs are most often observed two weeks after injury occurs (*Figures 10.3* and *10.4*). These include:
- slight stiffness of gait
- prolapse of the third eyelid which may cover as much as half the eye
- very erect and rigid ears
- a raised tail head
- a worried expression, with retraction of the eyelids and flaring nostrils due to spasm of the face muscles
- inability to open the mouth due to spasm in the masseter (chewing) muscles, hence the alternative name, lockjaw
- regurgitation of food and water from the nostrils and drooling of saliva from the mouth as swallowing becomes difficult.

As the disease progresses there is:
- rigid extension of the limbs, causing difficulty in moving
- progressive stiffness and extension of the neck
- rapid, shallow respiration
- muscle spasm or convulsions when stimulated by light, noise or touch
- urine and faecal retention
- inability to rise after falling over.

If left untreated, the animal will die from inhalation pneumonia (caused by food material and saliva entering the lungs) or from dehydration and malnutrition.

Treatment

This is rarely undertaken due to the very poor

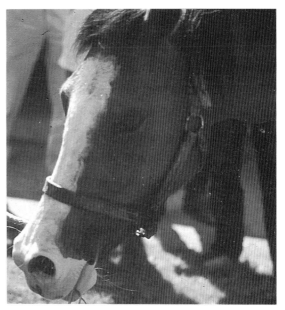

Figure 10.4   *Tetanus: this pony has flared nostrils and unchewed hay held in its 'locked' jaw*

prognosis and the costs involved. Where the horse is unable to rise, euthanasia is the kindest course of action.

Animals diagnosed in the very early stages of the disease have a greater chance of recovery, although they may require weeks or months of therapy and nursing.

Treatment includes:
- cleaning and removal of all scabs and dead tissue from the wound
- large doses of penicillin and tetanus antitoxin
- sedatives, e.g. acepromazine, to control anxiety and muscle spasms.

Feeding

Water and gruel may be given either by stomach tube or through a tube sutured directly into the oesophagus. When the horse can swallow, soft, palatable food should be offered. Feed and water containers must be raised to a suitable height.

Nursing

Patients should be nursed in familiar surroundings by their owners. Use a quiet, dark stable with a deep bed of woodshavings (straw tends to wind around the horse's legs). Establish a quiet and efficient nursing routine which disturbs the horse as little as possible.

Prevention

The risk of tetanus is greatly reduced if horses are regularly vaccinated with tetanus toxoid. This can be given in conjunction with the influenza vaccine (see Chapter 1).

Unvaccinated horses with wounds must be given tetanus antitoxin for immediate short term protection. When given early enough, it neutralises the toxin before it reaches the nervous system. *It is no substitute for full vaccination, which should be started at the same time.*

11 Physiotherapy

Physiotherapy

The purpose of physiotherapy is to assist natural healing of the tissues and to help restore normal function to the injured part of the body. It also provides pain relief and relaxation.

When tissue is damaged, the blood flow is disrupted. Excess fluid accumulates and causes swelling. Small veins become compressed and venous return of blood to the heart is impeded. Lack of muscular activity during the period of enforced rest compromises the circulation even more.

Faradic treatment

A portable machine produces an intermittent, alternating electrical current. When the faradic stimulator is applied to a muscle, it stimulates it to contract. The strength and duration of the current pulses can be altered. The benefits of this treatment include:
- toning up and gradual strengthening of weak muscles
- improved circulation which disperses inflammatory fluids and removes the waste products of muscle metabolism
- prevents muscle wasting
- helps to prevent the formation of adhesions.

Faradism can also be used to locate sore muscle groups in the horse's back, loins and quarters. As the injured muscle is stimulated, the horse shows signs of resentment and discomfort.

Once the painful muscles have been identified, the current is reduced, and the weaker contractions are used to assist the healing process.

Ultrasound

An ultrasound machine converts electrical energy into high frequency sound waves. These penetrate deep into the tissues and produce minute vibrations and heat.

Ultrasound is used for injuries to muscles, tendons and ligaments. The heat reduces muscle spasm and increases blood flow. Ultrasound also increases the elasticity of scar tissue.

The ultrasound machine should only be used by an experienced operator and never in doses higher or longer than recommended. Incorrectly used, it can cause bone damage.

Magnetic field therapy

These units produce a pulsed magnetic field. When applied to damaged tissue an electric current is produced. This is known to affect ion exchange across cell membranes; how this promotes healing is not fully understood. Magnetic field therapy stimulates the circulation in damaged tissue.

It is used on:
- fractures
- arthritic joints
- epiphysitis and splints
- sore shins
- tendon strains and bruises
- strained muscles and ligaments.

Laser treatment

The laser emits a beam of light which is absorbed by tissues. It stimulates the production of collagen which speeds up the healing process. Laser treatment has a pain relieving effect. It is used for:
- tendon, ligament and muscle injuries
- splints, sore shins
- surgical wounds
- open wounds
- control of proud flesh.

Electrostimulation

These machines use a low-energy electric current to stimulate healing. They are used for:
- tendon, ligament and muscle injuries
- sore shins and splints
- swollen joints
- arthritis
- fractures
- open wounds.

Comment

More research is needed for a better understanding of the effects of magnetic fields, laser treatment and electrical stimulation on the tissues. *The machines should be used only by experienced operators as incorrect use can be harmful.*

Massage

Massage can reduce swelling by assisting venous return. With the aid of a lubricant gel or massage oil, the tissues are massaged towards the heart.

Water currents can be used to massage the limbs. Special jacuzzi tubs and aqua boots have been developed for this purpose.

Exercise

Controlled exercise is a very important part of the rehabilitation programme following an injury. It improves venous flow and lymph drainage. It also reduces the chances of adhesions forming between individual tissues.

It is essential that the demands on the horse are increased very slowly to avoid the possibility of reinjury. A programme should be designed to develop suppleness and balance, while gradually building up muscular strength.

Exercise programmes begin with walking in hand and may work up to exercises over poles. The fitness requirements of the horse will be considered when the programme is devised.

Swimming

Swimming is useful in the early stages of the rehabilitation programme. It improves muscle tone and works the heart without the legs bearing weight or being subjected to concussion.

Swimming therapy should only be carried out under the direction of a physiotherapist. It is strenuous exercise and if the horse becomes exhausted, no benefit will be derived. Facilities for drying the horse must be available.

Heat treatment

Heat treatment is often used in conjunction with massage and controlled exercise. It should not be used within the first 24–48 hours after an injury occurs as it can provoke further haemorrhage.

Heat increases the blood supply to the damaged tissue. This provides increased oxygen and more white blood cells to clear up the debris. The improved blood and lymph flow promotes resorption of blood and fluid from the damaged tissue.

The warmth helps relieve muscle spasm and reduce the pain, making the horse more comfortable and relaxed.

Superficial heat

Superficial heat does not penetrate far beneath the skin. It can be applied by:
- heat lamps
- heated pads or blankets
- hot poultices
- hot tubbing.

Deep heat

Deep heat is provided by ultrasound.

Cold treatment

Cold treatment is used for bruises and strains of tendons, muscles, joints and ligaments. It is of maximum benefit immediately after the injury occurs and in the following 24–48 hours. With the exception of the initial hosing, it is not used for open wounds.

The coldness causes constriction of small arteries (arterioles). This decreases the amount of haemorrhage and swelling in the damaged tissue; it also helps to relieve pain.

As soon as the application of cold is withdrawn, the blood vessels dilate. In order to minimise the subsequent swelling, a support bandage should be applied to the injured area.

Cold can be applied in several ways:

Cold hosing

This should be done for 20 minutes three times a day.

Iced water

The affected limb is immersed in a bucket of very cold water. The treatment is done for 15 minutes three times a day.

Standing the horse in a stream is a very effective way of giving cold treatment. The specially designed aqua boot also provides underwater massage.

Frozen Gamgee

Wet Gamgee is frozen in the deep freeze. It is then roughly shaped and bandaged to the affected part. It stays cold for approximately 15 minutes.

Crushed ice, frozen peas

These are transferred to a polythene bag and bandaged on the injured area over a thin layer of Gamgee. Frozen substances must never be placed in direct contact with the skin or ice scald may occur. These may be left on for approximately 30 minutes.

Bonner bandages

These commercially available bandages pro

vide both cold and support. The bandage stays cold for 15 minutes after removal from the freezer.

Commercially produced gel packs

Flexible plastic sachets containing a gel are placed in the freezer for one and a half hours. The gel cools but does not freeze. The pack is applied over a layer of Gamgee and held in position by a stable bandage. It can be left on for two hours.

These packs can also be used for heat treatment. The sachet is immersed in warm water and applied as above. The gel retains the heat for several hours.

Alternate hot and cold treatment

Alternate hot and cold treatment is sometimes used to stimulate the circulation with an injury such as a sprain. Cold treatment alone is given for the first 24 hours, followed by 15 minute periods of alternate hot and cold treatments, each lasting 3–5 minutes, two or three times a day.

Topical pastes, gels and liniments

There are a large number of preparations on the market that claim to reduce swelling. They come in the form of cooling lotions, liniments, astringent gels and pastes.

Some are undoubtedly more effective than others. In many instances, as much benefit may be derived from the massage during application as from the product itself.

These preparations should not be applied to broken skin or open wounds.

If you need advice – consult your vet.

Blisters

Blistering agents cause acute inflammation and soreness of the skin. They are not recommended.

12 The Digestive System

Digestion

The digestive tract of the horse is designed to cope with the digestion of protein, fat and carbohydrates. In addition, the large intestine acts as a fermentation vat where bacteria and protozoa break down the cellulose component of grass, hay and grain (*Figure 12.1*).

Stages of digestion

Mouth

Food in the mouth is thoroughly chewed and mixed with saliva. The mucus content of saliva lubricates the passage of food down the oesophagus into the stomach. When food material becomes lodged in the oesophagus, it causes the condition known as *choke*.

The teeth must be kept in good order so that food material is sufficiently broken down before entering the stomach.

Stomach

Bacterial fermentation begins in the upper part of the stomach. As the food approaches the pylorus, the stomach contents become more acid and enzymes begin protein digestion.

The stomach of the horse is relatively small, with a capacity of some 7 to 8 litres. The horse should therefore be fed little and often to avoid digestive upsets.

Horses rarely vomit because there is a powerful muscular sphincter between the stomach and the lower end of the oesophagus. Food reflux occurs only when very high pressure builds up in the stomach. This can occur in horses with *grass sickness* and high *small intestinal obstructions*.

Small intestine (duodenum, jejunum, ileum)

The food passes out of the stomach into the duodenum, where it is mixed with pancreatic juice and bile. The digestive enzymes break down protein, carbohydrate and fat. Digestion and absorption occur along the length of the small intestine, which is approximately 21 metres.

The food material is moved along by contraction of smooth muscle in the gut wall. The waves of muscular activity are called peristalsis.

Large intestine (caecum, colon)

Undigested food and fibre now enter the large intestine where bacteria and protozoa continue the digestion of protein, carbohydrate and fat.

They also:
• ferment and digest cellulose

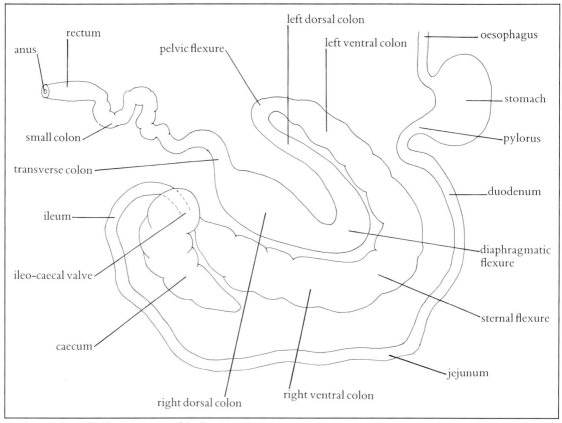

Figure 12.1   *The digestive tract of the horse*

- form essential amino acids
- produce B vitamins and vitamin K_2.

The bacterial population varies according to the nature of the diet – horses fed on hay and grass have different bacteria to those on high-concentrate diets. If the diet is suddenly changed, the fermentation process is disrupted and the horse may suffer from *colic*, *constipation* or *diarrhoea*.

In order to avoid such problems, changes to the diet should be made slowly over a period of two weeks. This allows the bacteria time to adapt to the different food.

Wild horses graze at regular intervals, whereas domesticated horses have their food intake controlled. This can lead to problems, especially if the horse eats large volumes of roughage in a short period of time. *Impactions* may develop at any of the three U-bends (known as flexures) in the large intestine.

Water is absorbed as the food passes through the large intestine.

Rectum

Undigested residues from the food eaten by the horse pass into the rectum and are expelled via the anus.

Choke

Choke occurs when food material obstructs the oesophagus.

Clinical signs

These include:
- coughing
- holding the head and neck in an extended position
- difficulty in swallowing; the horse flexes and then stretches the neck, often squealing or grunting in pain
- trickling of green or brown fluid or food from both nostrils
- saliva drooling from the mouth.

Causes

- Bolting of food: greedy, tired or anxious horses may swallow food before it is adequately chewed.
- Sharp teeth or a sore mouth may prevent normal chewing.
- Cubes and odd-shaped lumps of food such as carrots and apples can become lodged in the oesophagus.
- Inadequately soaked sugar beet can impact the oesophagus.

Immediate action

- Do not panic.
- Move the animal to a stable.
- Do not offer any food or water.
- Keep the horse under observation.

Many cases of choke clear spontaneously and do not require veterinary attention.

When the horse is very distressed or the condition has not resolved after 5–10 minutes, call the vet.

Treatment

The vet administers a tranquillizer and a drug to reduce the spasm of the oesophageal wall.

A stomach tube is sometimes passed to relieve the obstruction.

Management of horses with un-relieved choke

- Provide inedible bedding such as wood shavings, paper or peat.
- Do not offer food but make sure water is available.
- Leave the horse as undisturbed as possible.

Most horses recover within 24 hours.

Possible complications

If the oesophagus is firmly impacted with sugar beet or the choke is unrelieved after 24 hours, the obstruction is removed by continuous irrigation with water through a stomach tube. In some cases this requires general anaesthesia.

Aftercare of the patient

Once the obstruction is relieved, the horse should be offered grass or a small, damp feed several times a day.

Nuts should be thoroughly soaked or avoided altogether for a few days.

Allow the horse to graze in preference to consuming large quantities of hay. Gradually reintroduce *soaked* hay after 48 hours.

Prevention

- Offer hay before feeding concentrates to greedy or hungry horses.
- Place a salt lick in the bottom of the manger; this slows down feed consumption.
- Avoid feeding nuts to habitual chokers.

- Damp all feeds.
- Inspect the teeth regularly.

When the horses in a field are fed at different times, they tend to bolt their feed. If possible, take the horse out of the field, so it can eat its feed without interference from other horses.

Colic

Colic is the name given to a variety of conditions in which the horse suffers abdominal pain (*Figure 12.2*). It can vary widely in severity. Prompt treatment minimises the horse's distress and allows early diagnosis of surgical cases.

Many horse owners fear the worst when their horse has colic. However, *most colics are not serious and the horse recovers without complications* if correctly treated.

Clinical signs

The earliest signs may include some or all of the following.

The horse may be:
- less enthusiastic about its feed than normal or not eating at all
- passing fewer droppings than normal
- quiet and lethargic
- looking around at its flanks, kicking at its belly, or pawing the ground.

As the pain increases, there may be:
- patchy sweating
- attempts to lie down or roll
- fast, shallow breathing that develops into blowing
- spasms of severe pain which cause violent rolling and groaning
- distension of the abdomen.

When to call the vet

If the horse exhibits anything more than mild abdominal discomfort for a few minutes, the vet should be called.

Even if the horse is better by the time the vet arrives, discussion of the case may help avoid future incidents.

Immediate action

- Stay calm and keep spectators away.
- While the signs are mild, keep the horse in a stable and ensure there is plenty of bedding.
- If the horse is lying down quietly, do not force it to get up. It will be in the position it finds most comfortable. Remove buckets and any other fixtures on which it might injure itself if it starts rolling.
- A *few minutes* of quiet walking may stop a horse with mild colic from rolling. *Do not* walk it to the point of exhaustion.
- When a horse is rolling violently and continually in a stable, it is likely to become cast. In these cases it is often safer to move it to a field or a manege but well away from hazards such as ditches and fences.

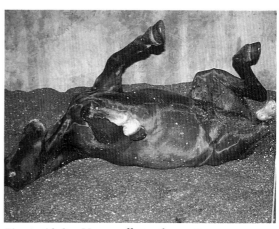

Figure 12.2   *Horse suffering from colic*

Note the following information for the vet:
- has the horse passed any droppings? If so, when and what consistency?
- are there any stomach rumbles and noises?
- is the pain intermittent or continuous?
- have there been any changes in the diet?

Do not:
- offer any food
- administer a colic drench; this could accidentally enter the lungs, with serious consequences.

Above all, *do not* risk injury to yourself or other people in your attempts to help the horse.

How to help the vet

- Make sure the horse is adequately restrained with a bridle or headcollar.
- Provide a bucket of warm water, soap and a towel.
- At night, have the horse in a well-lit stable when the vet arrives. Examination is more difficult when carried out by torch or car headlights.

The examination

The vet will carry out a thorough examination of the horse. This serves two purposes.

Firstly, to establish whether the horse really has colic or whether it is suffering from some other condition causing colic-like symptoms. Amongst the more common false colics are:
- laminitis
- azoturia
- foaling
- uterine rupture and haemorrhage.

Secondly, the examination and history will sometimes reveal the cause of the abdominal pain. Specific treatments may then be pre-scribed. The examination includes the following tests.

Taking the pulse and temperature

The pulse rises in response to pain and cardiovascular shock.

With spasmodic colic, the pulse may rise as high as 90 during the bouts of pain, but then return close to normal. A pulse that remains above 60 in the quiet periods despite the administration of analgesics is of more concern.

Checking gut activity

The vet will listen to the chest and abdomen with a stethoscope to establish whether the gut activity is greater or less than normal.

Observation of the respiratory pattern

Fast, shallow breathing often accompanies severe colic.

Examination of the mucous membranes

The gums of a healthy horse are a pale salmon pink colour.

In a serious colic they change colour, becoming redder, bluish purple or greyish white. The conjunctival membranes turn from salmon pink to brick red as circulatory difficulties are experienced.

Measurement of capillary refill time

Pressing firmly on the horse's gum blanches the mucous membrane. The pink colour should return within three seconds – failure to do so indicates cardiovascular shock.

Rectal examination

(Under no circumstances should this test – or the three which follow it – be attempted by anyone other than a vet.)

Much valuable information can be obtained from examining the horse per rectum. The vet will feel for:

- droppings in the rectum, to see if food material is still passing through the horse. The consistency is checked for evidence of diarrhoea or constipation
- impaction of the large bowel
- loops of intestine distended by gas
- evidence of redworm damage to the blood supply of the gut
- tight bands of tissue and sites of acute pain indicating bowel displacement.

With a severe twist, the rectum may be so tight that internal examination is not possible.

Other procedures that may be carried out include:

Passing a stomach tube

A warm and flexible stomach tube is passed up the horse's nostril, into the pharynx. When the horse swallows, the tube is pushed down the oesophagus, into the stomach.

This procedure may help to establish a diagnosis. For example, release of a large amount of gas and fluid suggests that the problem lies in the stomach or the first part of the small intestine. The stomach tube is also used to administer some treatments, e.g. liquid paraffin (*Figure 12.3*).

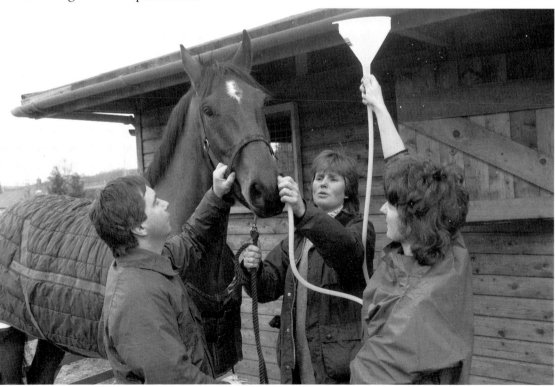

Figure 12.3   *Liquid paraffin and saline are given by stomach tube to horses with impactions*

Blood tests

Where the cause of colic is unclear, a blood sample may be taken as an aid to diagnosis. In certain cases, the vet will monitor the horse's 'packed cell volume' (PCV) (see Chapter 19). Results of 45 or more indicate circulatory disturbance. The higher the PCV, the graver the prognosis.

Peritoneal tap

This test involves collecting a small sample of fluid from the horse's abdominal cavity. The lowest part of the abdomen is clipped and scrubbed and a needle is inserted through the ventral midline. A fluid sample is collected.

Normal peritoneal fluid is a clear pale straw colour. If the horse has an infection of the abdomen (peritonitis), the fluid is cloudy. A ruptured gut may yield brownish fluid with visible vegetable matter. This test is carried out as a routine aid to diagnosis or when complications are suspected.

Types of colic and their causes

In the following sections, brief descriptions of the types of colic most commonly treated in practice are given. For descriptive purposes they can be divided into medical or surgical colics.

Medical Colics

Medical colics can be divided into four main types: gastric, spasmodic and tympanitic colic, and food impactions.

Gastric colic

As the horse's stomach is small in size, it is prone to overdistension. This may be caused by:
- food, e.g. gorging of unsoaked sugar beet, which then expands
- gas, e.g. grass cuttings and apples ferment after being eaten, creating large volumes of gas in the stomach.

Spasmodic colic

Spasmodic colic occurs when the smooth pattern of peristalsis is disrupted. The peristaltic movements become violent and irregular – the horse shows periods of acute pain interspersed with periods of calm.

Causes include:
- damage to the intestinal blood supply by redworm larvae
- sudden change in diet
- irregular feeding
- fatigue and/or anxiety.

Tympanitic colic

Unsuitable food, e.g. grass cuttings, clover and apples, leads to abnormal fermentation and accumulation of gas in the intestine.

There may be visible abdominal distension and the pain is likely to be very severe. The gas-filled intestine is more liable to twist than normal, therefore when this type of colic is suspected from the history of the case, you should try to stop the horse from rolling.

Food impactions

At grass, the horse grazes for many hours of the day so food passes through the gut at a steady rate. The stabled horse has its diet artificially regulated and impactions may develop. The pelvic flexure is the commonest site of impaction because the gut narrows and turns through 180 degrees at this site.

Other factors which may play a part in the development of impactions include:
- redworm damage affecting the normal motility of the gut
- neglected teeth
- unsuitable diet
- bed eating
- insufficient access to water
- change in management, e.g. box rest.

In the early stages the pain is less acute than in the other types of colic described. The horse may:
- adopt a urinating stance and strain intermittently
- walk backwards into the corner of the box
- lie flat out or sit up and look round at its flanks
- get up and down, stamp its feet and occasionally roll.

Treatment of medical colics

Each case of colic is treated individually, taking into account the history, the clinical signs, and any other relevant information.
The aims of the treatment are:
- pain relief
- elimination of the cause of discomfort
- prevention of secondary problems, e.g. infection.

Treatment may include:

Analgesia

Analgesics are administered to all cases of colic. Some have a relaxing effect on the muscle of the gut wall and help to re-establish normal peristalsis.

Sedatives

These help to reduce anxiety and slow down gut movement.

Liquid paraffin and saline

Large quantities are given by stomach tube to horses with an impaction. The mixture helps to break up the mass of accumulated material.

Anti-fermentative drugs

Oil of turpentine, for example, may be given with liquid paraffin to a horse with tympanitic colic.
Passing the stomach tube may in itself give relief as it allows gas to escape, so relieving pressure on the stomach.

Anthelmintics

These are given where worms are suspected as the cause of the colic.

Antibiotics

Antibiotics are given at the discretion of the vet, depending upon the clinical and laboratory findings.

Care of the patient

Your vet will advise on:
- feeding, including grazing
- exercise and return to work
- prevention of further attacks.

Surgical Colics

Horses with this type of colic will not recover without surgery. For a variety of reasons a portion of gut is deprived of its blood supply and dies. This is known as *infarction*.

The normally pink intestine goes through a series of colour changes from red to bluish-black and finally grey-green. Bacterial poisons, called toxins, leak out through the damaged gut wall and the horse shows signs of extreme shock. Unless surgery is carried out promptly, the horse will die.

Causes

Causes of infarction include:

Redworm damage

Larvae of *Strongylus vulgaris* damage the lining of the main artery supplying the gut.

Blood clots, called emboli, break away from the lining and are released into the blood-stream. They can block small vessels and cause thromboembolic colic.

There are two possible consequences:

- there may be mild, transient colic due to partial occlusion of small vessels. The reduced blood supply causes the normal pattern of peristalsis to change
- the gut may not recover and can undergo infarction. If just a short segment of small intestine is involved, the horse may be saved by surgical removal of the affected piece of gut. When a number of emboli block several vessels, the prognosis is hopeless.

Intussusception

This is most common in foals and yearlings. A piece of intestine becomes folded inside an adjacent piece of gut, causing a partial or total obstruction. This is often due to heavy ascarid worm burdens or redworm damage which interfere with normal gut motility.

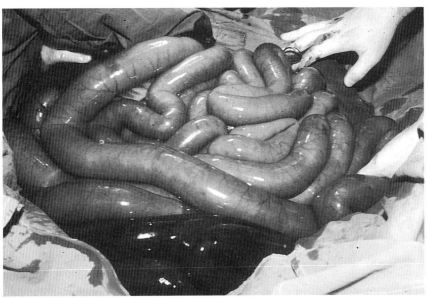

Figure 12.4
Pony undergoing colic surgery. The strangulated intestine in the foreground was removed and the pony recovered

Twist of the small or large intestine

The small intestine can spontaneously form knots, and the large bowel can twist upon itself.

In each case the blood supply is stopped, leading to infarction.

Strangulation by pedunculated lipomas

In older animals, benign, fatty tumours may be found attached to the mesentery by string-like lengths of tissue. These can wind around a piece of small intestine, blocking the passage of food, and occluding the blood supply.

Surgery or euthanasia?

When a surgical colic is diagnosed, the horse should be operated on as quickly as possible or humanely destroyed.

This is never an easy decision. Be guided by your vet; some abdominal crises occur so quickly that by the time the horse is examined, surgery is no longer a realistic option.

Some of the factors that must be considered include:

Distance to the nearest operating facilities

The sooner surgery commences, the greater the chance of a successful outcome. It is kinder to destroy the horse than subject it to a long and pointless journey.

The age of the horse or pony

Older animals should be operated on only if they are likely to overcome the trauma.

The financial implications

Colic surgery requires three vets for a period of several hours. The intensive care and fluid therapy that follows is also expensive and the total cost is likely to be in excess of £1,000.

Chance of survival

Only about one in four horses survive colic surgery. This is because many cases are found to be inoperable when the gut is examined and the horse is euthanased on the operating table.

Prevention of Colic

The risk of colic occurring can be reduced by sensible management.
- Worm your horse every 4–6 weeks.
- Use only fresh, good quality feed; throw away anything mouldy or suspect.
- Do not work the horse for at least an hour after feeding, or feed immediately after strenuous work.
- Make any changes to the feeding regime over a period of two weeks.
- Know your horse, so you can tell if it is off colour: if in doubt, keep it under close observation.

Liver Disease

The liver has many functions.

These include:
- production of bile
- regulation of blood sugar levels
- breakdown of excess protein to urea (excreted by the kidneys)
- metabolism of fats
- synthesis of blood clotting factors
- production of blood proteins
- detoxification of poisonous compounds.

Causes

The causes of liver disease include:
- plant toxins, e.g. ragwort
- viruses
- bacteria
- tumours
- severe energy deficiency
- chemical toxins, e.g. arsenic or phosphorus.

When damaged, the liver has enormous capacity for regeneration. When this capacity is exceeded, the damaged cells are replaced by non-functional fibrous tissue. Symptoms develop when there are insufficient healthy cells to cope with the functions listed above.

Clinical signs

The clinical signs are extremely variable and develop over a period of time. Some of the following will be apparent:
- weight loss
- lack of appetite
- staring coat
- abdominal pain
- diarrhoea
- photosensitisation of non-pigmented skin
- fluid collection under the skin of the belly (ventral oedema)
- jaundice

Behavioural signs include:
- depression
- sleepiness
- excessive yawning
- restlessness and aimless wandering.

In the advanced stages of the disease there may be:
- circling
- head pressing against solid objects
- blindness
- incoordination
- excitement
- maniacal behaviour
- coma.

Diagnosis

Diagnosis is made on clinical signs and the results of blood tests. A liver biopsy may yield further information on the cause and extent of the disease.

Treatment

There is no specific treatment. All therapy is aimed at supporting the liver, in the hope that cell regeneration will occur.
This supportive treatment includes:
- high energy, low protein diet
- glucose by mouth or intravenously
- B vitamins
- antibiotics
- complete rest.

The disease is monitored by regular blood tests.

Prognosis

The prognosis is always guarded. Horses that have apparently recovered often relapse as soon as they go back into work.
Once the terminal stages have been reached, the horse may behave in a dangerous manner and should be humanely destroyed.

Hyperlipaemia

This is a condition where an abnormal amount of fat accumulates in the blood. It occurs in animals which have insufficient food to meet their energy requirements.

To compensate, fat is mobilised from stores in the body. The liver uses some of this fat to produce energy. However, if the period of energy deficiency is prolonged, the liver and bloodstream become overloaded with fat and symptoms develop.

Small, fat ponies and cobs are especially susceptible. Hyperlipaemia is most commonly seen in mares that are inadequately fed in late pregnancy and early lactation.

Causes

The major causes of hyperlipaemia are stress and insufficient food intake.

Typical stress factors include:
- pregnancy
- lactation
- transportation
- heavy worm burden
- any disease causing inappetance
- drastic starvation of laminitic ponies.

Clinical signs

Affected animals are usually dull and lethargic. They show little interest in food or their

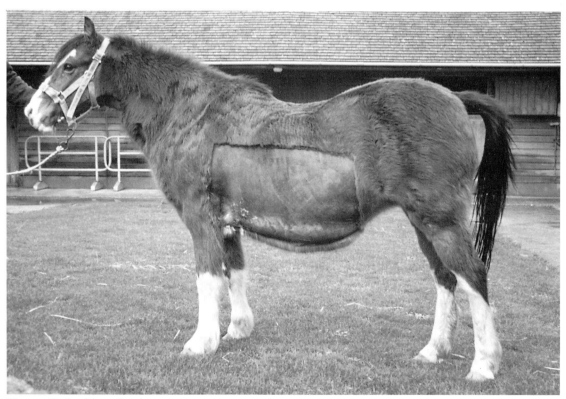

Figure 12.5   *Ventral oedema in a pony mare with hyperlipaemia. (The abdomen has been clipped)*

surroundings. They frequently stand over the trough and play with water without drinking. There is rapid loss of condition. Abdominal pain is experienced as a result of swelling of the liver.

Other possible symptoms include fever, jaundice and ventral oedema (*Figure 12.5*). Fatty, foul-smelling diarrhoea may be produced in the terminal stages.

Diagnosis

Diagnosis is confirmed by taking a blood sample. The plasma looks milky instead of the normal clear yellow colour. Blood tests are carried out to assess the degree of liver damage.

Treatment

Early diagnosis is essential for treatment to have any chance of success. Most ponies with hyperlipaemia do not recover.

The most important considerations are:
• reducing stress
• increasing the energy intake.

Reducing stress

Stress is reduced by immediate treatment of any other condition. Aborting a pregnant mare may increase her chances of survival. The stress of lactation can be reduced by early weaning of the foal.

Increasing the energy intake

Increasing the energy intake prevents further quantities of fat being mobilised into the bloodstream. Every effort should be made to encourage the pony to eat. Offer a choice of foods and let the pony select its favourite. Affected ponies often prefer fresh green grass to anything else.

If the pony will not eat, glucose can be mixed with a high-energy gruel and administered by stomach tube.

Medication

Insulin is given by injection.

Heparin is sometimes used as it speeds up the rate of fat removal from the blood. However, this drug delays the clotting time of blood which must therefore be closely monitored throughout treatment.

Prevention

Ensure that the energy intake of susceptible animals is adequate at all times of the year.

Broodmares considered to be at risk should have regular blood tests in late pregnancy and early to peak lactation. The plasma begins to look milky before the pony becomes noticeably ill.

If in doubt, seek veterinary advice on the nutrition of pregnant mares. If mares are being transported long distances to and from a stud, stop regularly and allow them to rest and eat.

Take care when restricting the diet of laminitic ponies. Drastic starvation is to be avoided.

Diarrhoea

Diarrhoea can be mild and self-limiting or serious and life-threatening. It may be accompanied by colicky pain.

Causes

The causes include:
- excitement/nervousness
- sudden dietary changes, e.g. access to lush grass, change of hay
- worms
- prolonged use of antibiotics which remove the normal gut flora
- infection by bacteria or viruses, e.g. Salmonella
- tumours
- poisoning.

When to call the vet

As diarrhoea is a symptom of many conditions, there are no hard and fast rules. The following guidelines are offered:
- if the horse is off colour or has a temperature, the vet should be called immediately
- if the horse seems fine in itself but has uncharacteristically loose droppings for more than a day or two, it should be seen by the vet
- *foals* with diarrhoea should be examined by the vet as soon as the condition is observed.

Diarrhoea due to excitement or sudden dietary change is usually transitory and requires sensible management rather than veterinary treatment.

Diagnosis

The first step with either acute or chronic diarrhoea is to try and find the cause through clinical examination and discussion of the history.
The vet may take:
- blood samples to check for evidence of infection or worm infestation
- dung samples to check for worm eggs and pathogenic bacteria and viruses

- a rectal biopsy and a sample of peritoneal fluid from the abdomen if tumours are suspected.

Treatment

Whatever the cause, the principles of treatment are the same. They include:
- removal of the cause
- fluid and electrolyte replacement
- the use of drugs which reduce the speed of food passage along the gut (allowing more time for water absorption)
- restoration of the normal population of gut microorganisms.

Management

Stable the horse.
Feed good quality hay – do not allow the horse to graze or consume any succulent feed such as carrots or sugar beet.
Allow water ad lib. If electrolytes are added, fresh water should also be available as some horses dislike the taste of electrolytes, and stop drinking. Horses with diarrhoea need to drink more than usual to replace the extra fluid lost. Restricting water can result in dehydration.
If an infectious cause is suspected, the horse must be isolated.

Medication

- If worms are diagnosed, dose with a suitable anthelmintic.
- Gut sedatives such as chlorodyne or codeine phosphate slow the passage of food through the gut.
- Spasmolytic and analgesic drugs relieve colicky pain.
- Oral administration of adsorbents, e.g. kaolin, aluminium hydroxide, activated

charcoal and bismuth subnitrate reduces absorption of toxins produced by pathogenic bacteria.
- Antibiotics are prescribed if the diarrhoea is caused by harmful bacteria.
- Feeding probiotics (preparations of normal gut bacteria) helps restore the normal balance of microorganisms which is disrupted when persistent diarrhoea occurs.
- Vitamin B may need supplementation as this is normally produced by gut bacteria.
- Large volumes of intravenous fluids may be needed in severe cases of diarrhoea.

Your vet will recommend the appropriate treatment after examining the horse.

Grass Sickness

Grass sickness is a disease in which degeneration of nerves leads to paralysis of the whole digestive tract from the pharynx to the rectum. It can affect horses of any age, but is most commonly seen in animals of 3–7 years.

The condition occurs in animals at grass. Horses recently turned out after winter stabling seem to be particularly at risk. The peak incidence is from April to July, especially during fine, dry spells. Certain fields are associated with an abnormally high incidence of the disease.

Cause

The cause is still unknown.

Clinical signs

These are variable, but will include some of

the following.

High pulse, sweating, muscular tremors

This will be accompanied by a rapid loss of condition.

Difficulty swallowing

Attempts to eat and drink are slow and clumsy. Chewed food and water may be dropped from the mouth or fall from the nostrils.

Thirsty horses that are unable to swallow stand over the trough and play with water. Saliva drools from the mouth.

Dehydration

The horse quickly becomes dehydrated and little urine is passed.

Stomach distension

The stomach may become so distended that its contents are forcibly regurgitated and run from both nostrils.

Reduced gut motility

Gut sounds are reduced or absent and the few droppings that are passed are small, hard and dry.

Abdominal pain

Horses with grass sickness experience abdo-

Figure 12.6   *Pony with chronic grass sickness. Note the tucked-up appearance, weight loss and clamped-down tail*

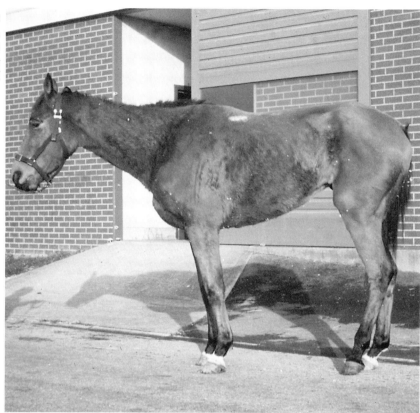

minal pain and may have episodes of severe colic.

Many animals adopt a typical stance. The head and neck are extended; all four feet are close together under the body and the tail is firmly clamped down (*Figure 12.6*).

Treatment

There is no cure. As soon as the condition is diagnosed the horse should be humanely destroyed.

Prognosis

The disease may be acute, subacute or chronic, but the end result is the same. Acute cases die in 1–4 days, subacute cases within three weeks while chronic cases may survive for weeks or months. The prognosis is therefore hopeless.

Prevention

Until the cause is established, it is difficult to suggest preventive measures. However, the disease has a high incidence in some parts of the country. Suspect fields should not be grazed by horses, especially during the spring and early summer. Hay cut from the field must not be fed to horses.

The cause of grass sickness may be a plant toxin. Cattle and sheep are not affected and should be introduced to eat the spring grass.

13 Poisonous Plants

Poisonous Plants

There are a large number of poisonous plants in Britain. Horses and ponies at pasture are often at risk, especially at those times of the year when grass is in short supply.

As far as possible, poisonous plants (*Figure 13.1*) should be identified and removed from the pasture. The effects of three of the most dangerous plants will now be described.

Ragwort (*Senecio jacobaea*)

Ragwort (*Figure 13.2*) contains alkaloids which cause irreversible liver damage. The characteristic yellow flowers are a common sight on horse-sick pastures.

The growing plant tastes very bitter and horses usually avoid it. However, once it is

Oak	St John's wort	Greater celandine
Ragwort	Bog asphodel	Corncockle
Yew	Pimpernel	Flax
Laburnum	Potato	Buckthorn
Hemlock	Iris	Alder buckthorn
Laurel	Henbane	Cowbane
Rhododendron	Lily of the valley	Hemlock water
Foxglove	Bulbs of: daffodil,	dropwort
Privet	hyacinth, snowdrop	Broom
Bracken	and bluebell	Hemp
Horsetail	Columbine	White bryony
Lupin	Hellebore	Thornapple
Poppy	Fritillaria	Sowbread
Buttercup	Soapwort	Meadow saffron
Chickweed	Sandwort	Herb paris
Deadly nightshade	Larkspur	Black bryony
Black nightshade	Monkshood	Darnel

Figure 13.1 *Poisonous plants found in Britain*

cut and dried, the plant becomes palatable. It is most dangerous when baled with hay.

Clinical signs

The effects of the alkaloid are cumulative and symptoms are not usually evident until a few weeks after the horse has been eating ragwort.

The signs of poisoning include any of the symptoms listed under Liver Disease (see Chapter 12), e.g.:

- anorexia and weight loss
- depression
- yawning
- abdominal pain
- constipation or diarrhoea
- head pressing against fixed objects
- circling and aimless walking
- collection of fluid under the skin of the belly
- jaundice
- incoordination.

In the terminal stages, the horse may go into a coma and die quietly or become delirious and suffer convulsions.

Treatment

There is no specific treatment. Supportive therapy is as described for Liver Disease (see page 129).

Prognosis

The prognosis is always guarded.

Prevention

Familiarise yourself with the appearance of ragwort and check the pasture regularly.

Pull up any plants and *remove* them from the field. The plant becomes palatable (and therefore dangerous) after treatment with a selective weed-killer.

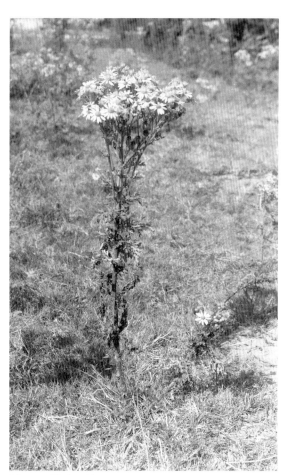

Figure 13.2 *Ragwort*

Yew (*Taxus baccata*)

All parts of the yew tree (*Figure 13.3*) are very poisonous. They contain the alkaloid taxine which has toxic effects on the heart. *One mouthful is enough to kill.*

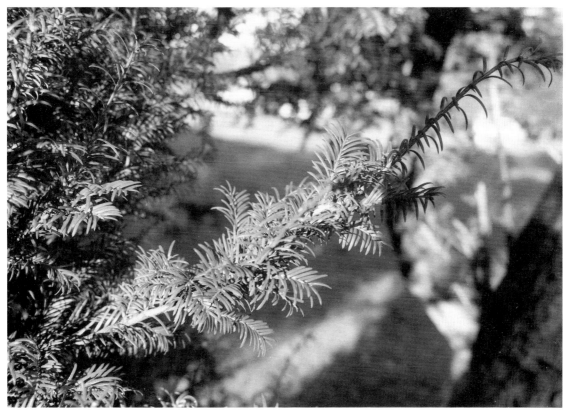

Figure 13.3   *Yew*

Clinical signs

Symptoms are rarely observed as the horse may die within five minutes of ingesting the poison. They include:
- muscular tremors
- staggering
- convulsions
- difficulty in breathing
- collapse
- heart failure.

Treatment

There is no antidote and no treatment.

Prevention

It is essential to check hedgerows for the presence of yew. When found, it should be fenced off or cut down.

Acorn Poisoning

Oak leaves and acorns contain tannic acid which is poisonous to horses.

Acorns are addictive; once a horse has acquired the taste, it will actively search for them. Oak poisoning causes gastroenteritis and kidney damage.

Clinical signs

These include:
- dullness
- loss of appetite
- abdominal pain
- constipation, followed by diarrhoea, which may be bloodstained
- blood in the urine.

Treatment

There is no antidote. The horse is treated with drugs to reduce the pain and control the diarrhoea. Antibiotics may be prescribed.

Prevention

Fence off oak trees – either permanently or with electric fencing.

Pick up all the fallen acorns at least once a day. This method is time-consuming and less effective as the horse will still find some.

How many acorns is it safe for a horse to eat?

Individual animals have different levels of tolerance. It is therefore impossible to say how many acorns can be eaten in a given period of time without causing symptoms.

However, what is certain is that horses and ponies die from acorn poisoning each autumn. The only way to keep the horse safe is to ensure that it has *no opportunity* to consume acorns or large quantities of foliage.

14 The Respiratory System

The Respiratory System

Breathing permits the exchange of oxygen and carbon dioxide between the tissues of the body and the air.

During inspiration, contraction of the diaphragm and the muscles between the ribs causes the chest cavity to expand and the lungs to fill with air.

When these muscles relax, air is exhaled. A slight contraction of the abdominal muscles helps push air from the lungs.

The normal respiratory rate is 8–16 breaths per minute.

The exchange of gases

Air enters the nostrils and passes along the nasal passages (*Figure 14.1*). It is drawn through the pharynx and larynx into the trachea.

The trachea runs down the underside of the neck and into the chest cavity where it divides into two bronchi (*Figure 14.2*).

The bronchi branch into progressively smaller tubes; the finest airways are called bronchioles.

Each bronchiole ends in a cluster of air sacs or alveoli. The thin, elastic walls of the air sacs are in close contact with a dense network of capillaries (*Figure 14.3*).

Capillaries are tiny, thin-walled blood vessels. Oxygen in the inhaled air diffuses from the air sac into the blood. It combines with haemoglobin in the red blood cells and is transported to the tissues. Carbon dioxide diffuses in the opposite direction and is exhaled.

During its passage from the nostrils to the lungs, air is warmed, moistened and filtered. Inhaled dust and spores are trapped by a thin layer of mucus which lines the airways. The mucus is continually moved towards the pharynx by tiny, hair-like projections on the epithelial cells. On reaching the pharynx, the debris is swallowed.

The effect of respiratory disease

When the horse succumbs to infectious or allergic respiratory disease, the quiet, relaxed pattern of breathing changes.

This is because the diameter of the airways is reduced by:
- excessive production of mucus or pus
- inflammation and swelling of the epithelial cells lining the airways
- spasm of smooth muscle in the airway walls.

Gas exchange is less efficient and more effort is needed to draw the same amount of air through the narrowed tubes. The smallest airways may become completely blocked.

Prompt treatment is required to prevent

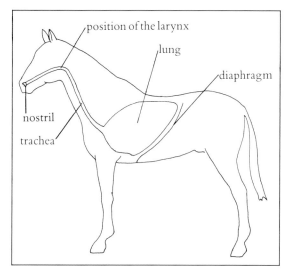

Figure 14.1   *The respiratory system of the horse*

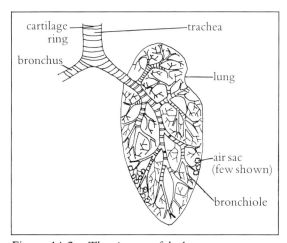

Figure 14.2   *The airways of the lung*

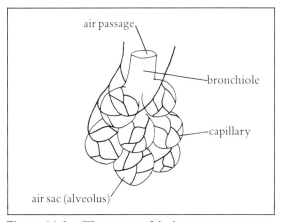

Figure 14.3   *The air sacs of the lung*

permanent damage occurring to the delicate lung tissues.

Diseases of the respiratory system include:
- viral infections
- bacterial infections
- parasitic infections
- allergic conditions.

Veterinary Examination

When you call the vet to examine a horse with respiratory disease, the consultation begins with a discussion of the horse's symptoms.

The vet will need information about the horse's management, including details of:
- diet
- type of bedding
- grazing and worming history
- vaccination status
- the type of work the horse does
- any recent exposure to respiratory disease, e.g. through attendance at shows.

The horse is given a thorough clinical examination which includes:
- observation of the rate and character of breathing while the horse is resting and relaxed
- taking the temperature
- listening to the chest with a stethoscope
- feeling for enlarged lymph nodes (glands)
- observation of any nasal discharge.

Where appropriate, samples will be taken for examination in the laboratory, e.g.:
- blood
- swabs
- faeces
- a tracheal wash.

In certain conditions the upper respiratory tract is examined with an endoscope.

Endoscopic Examination

The fibreoptic endoscope is used for visual examination of the upper respiratory tract (*Figure 14.4*).

Procedure

A long, flexible tube is passed into one nostril, along the nasal passages and into the pharynx.

Light is conducted along the glass fibres to the end of the instrument and illuminates the surrounding tissue. The tip of the endoscope can be moved in one or two planes. A clear, bright picture is transmitted back to the eyepiece.

The larynx is viewed from the nasopharynx. The endoscope can then be pushed through the laryngeal opening into the trachea and passed as far as the division into the two main bronchi.

There is usually very little resentment of this procedure. The horse is restrained in a stable with a headcollar and twitch.

Tracheal wash

The endoscope can also be used to obtain tracheal wash samples.

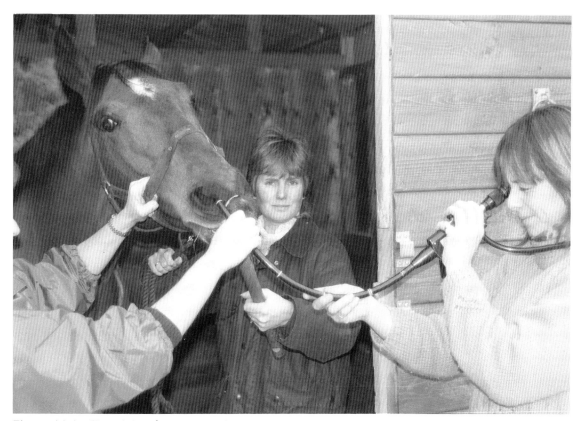

Figure 14.4 *Examining the upper respiratory tract with an endoscope*

Procedure

A long, sterile catheter is passed through a channel in the instrument and 20–50 ml of sterile saline is injected.

The saline runs down the wall of the trachea and washes epithelial cells, white (or occasionally red) blood cells and bacteria from the lining of the airway. The fluid collects at the entrance to the chest cavity and is sucked back up the catheter.

Bacteriological culture and microscopic examination of the tracheal wash sample can be an important aid to diagnosis. For example:
- the wash from a horse with pneumonia usually has large numbers of neutrophils and pathogenic bacteria. Antibiotic sensitivity tests performed on the bacterial cultures help the vet to select an antibiotic that will kill the bacteria
- abnormally high numbers of eosinophils may be seen if the horse has lungworm. Lungworm larvae are occasionally seen in the wash.

Equine Influenza

Equine influenza is a very infectious disease. It is caused by several strains of influenza virus and spreads rapidly through groups of horses.

The incubation period is 1–3 days.

Clinical signs

These include:
- a temperature of 39–41 °C (103–106 °F) which lasts 1–4 days
- watery nasal discharge which may rapidly become purulent
- a harsh, dry cough
- enlarged glands under the lower jaw
- conjunctivitis
- depression
- loss of appetite.

The symptoms persist for 1–3 weeks. Vaccinated horses may suffer a milder form of the disease.

When to call the vet

Consult the vet whenever your horse is coughing or has a temperature.

Diagnosis

Diagnosis is made on:
- clinical signs
- isolation of virus from nasopharyngeal swabs
- rising antibody levels in blood samples taken early in the course of the disease and 2–3 weeks later
- history of recent contact with confirmed cases of the disease.

Treatment

Horses with respiratory infections require:

Plenty of fresh air

The stable must be well ventilated. If weather conditions permit, affected horses benefit from being turned out for at least part of the day once their temperatures have subsided. This is especially important in the recovery stages.

Freedom from dust and spores

Exposure to dust and moulds should be minimised as horses with respiratory infections are prone to developing chronic obstructive pulmonary disease (COPD).

All hay should be soaked.

Complete rest

The horse must be rested for two weeks after the symptoms have disappeared.

Medication

The following drugs may be prescribed:
- antibiotics are given if
  - the nasal discharge becomes thick and yellow, indicating secondary bacterial infection
  - blood tests show evidence of secondary bacterial infection
- mucolytic drugs reduce the viscosity of the mucus
- bronchodilators relieve spasm of smooth muscle in the walls of the airways.

No antiviral drugs are available.

Control

The disease is spread by:
- inhalation of droplets released during coughing
- ingestion of discharges on shared tack, buckets and handler's clothing.

Strict hygiene and isolation procedures should be enforced (see Strangles, this chapter). Apparently healthy horses in an infected yard should not attend shows, etc., as they may be incubating the disease.

Complications

Problems are more likely to occur if the horse is given insufficient rest before resuming work. Complications include:
- COPD
- pneumonia – young foals are particularly at risk
- heart disease
- liver disease
- anaemia.

Prevention

- Establish a regular vaccination programme for *every horse* in the yard. Do not overlook youngstock, donkeys and elderly companions.
- Boost the immunity of pregnant mares a month *before* foaling to give maximum protection to the foal.
- In the event of an epidemic *do not* attend shows or any other equine gathering.

When an outbreak of equine influenza occurs, it is recommended that any horse which has not been vaccinated in the previous 4–6 months is given a booster.

Vaccines must only be given to healthy horses. Animals that are, or have recently been in contact with horses suffering from influenza should not be vaccinated as they may already be incubating the disease.

N.B. The horse does not gain maximum immunity until two weeks after receiving a booster injection.

Equine Herpes Virus 1

There are two subtypes of equine herpes virus 1 (EHV–1).

- Subtype 1 – which is also known as EHV–1, abortion strain.
- Subtype 2 – also known as EHV–4, respiratory strain.

For descriptive purposes they will be referred to as EHV–1 and EHV–4. Both subtypes are a common cause of respiratory disease in foals and yearlings.

Clinical signs

The following symptoms are common to both EHV–1 and EHV–4:
- high temperature, up to 41 °C (106 °F)
- swollen glands
- depression and lethargy
- loss of appetite
- watery nasal discharge which becomes purulent if secondary bacterial infection occurs
- occasional coughing (more frequent in young animals).

Additional symptoms associated with EHV–1 include:
- oedema (swelling) of the throat, neck and lower limbs
- abortion, mainly between 8–11 months, but it may occur any time from five months onwards
- the birth of weak, jaundiced foals that usually die in the first week
- incoordination/paralysis; dribbling urine is an early sign of the paralytic form.

Viral abortion

EHV–1 infection does not always cause abortion in pregnant mares. It is more likely to cross the placenta and infect the fetus than EHV–4. It sometimes causes multiple abortions on a stud, whereas EHV–4 results in the occasional single abortion. When a mare does abort, it may be 7–10 days after infection or several months later.

Transmission is by inhalation of virus released into the atmosphere from the respiratory tract of infected animals or from aborted material. It is possible for a horse to carry and spread the virus without showing any symptoms.

When to call the vet

Consult the vet as soon as the horse shows any of the symptoms listed.

Diagnosis

Clinical examination alone does not distinguish between the two subtypes or other viruses affecting the upper respiratory tract. Diagnosis is therefore made on:
- culture of the virus from
  - nasopharyngeal swabs taken early in the course of the disease
  - blood and fresh tissues from the aborted fetus, dead foal or paralysed horse (following euthanasia).
- measurement of antibody levels in the blood. As soon as a horse is challenged by the virus, antibody levels begin to rise. Blood is taken when the symptoms first appear and three weeks later. A marked rise in antibodies indicates recent infection. A high reading from a single blood test is also a sign of recent exposure to the virus.
- postmortem findings and microscopic examination of tissues from the aborted fetus or foal.

Treatment

Treatment of the respiratory symptoms is as described for equine influenza, i.e.:
- fresh air
- complete rest

- antibiotics, mucolytics and bronchodilators as necessary.

Horses showing incoordination or paralysis are treated with anti-inflammatory drugs, intravenous fluids and careful nursing. In severe cases, euthanasia is necessary.

There is no specific treatment for mares following abortion. Isolation is essential as the mare may shed virus for a considerable period of time.

Control measures

Vaccination

Pregnant mares may be vaccinated during months five, seven and nine of the pregnancy. The immunity following vaccination and natural infection is poor, lasting only 2–3 months.

The vaccine will not prevent an individual abortion in the face of a heavy disease challenge. However, vaccination of all the mares on the premises reduces shedding of the virus from infected individuals and may help to prevent a storm of abortions occurring.

Horses in contact with pregnant mares may be given two doses of vaccine, 3–4 weeks apart. A booster is given six months later and then annually.

Course of action when a mare aborts

Whenever a mare aborts or a foal dies within 10 days of birth, the cause should be investigated. Early detection of EHV–1 is especially important if the mare is in contact with other pregnant mares. If the situation arises:
- contact the vet immediately
- isolate the mare in a stable
- put the fetus and membranes in a leak-proof container
- disinfect any areas likely to be contaminated by fetal fluids.

A Code of Practice has been drawn up by the Thoroughbred Breeders' Association to minimise the spread of infectious reproductive disease. It offers guidelines on all aspects of prevention and control of the disease. The recommendations include the following:
- the fetus and membranes should be sent to a laboratory for examination
- in-contact mares should be managed as though infected until the results are available
- no horses should be moved onto or off the premises until EHV–1 infection has been ruled out.

The vet will advise you of the disinfection procedure and answer any queries you may have.

Strangles

Strangles is a highly infectious and contagious disease affecting the upper respiratory tract of horses. It is caused by the bacterium *Streptococcus equi*.

It affects horses of all ages but young animals are particularly susceptible. The incubation period is 3–8 days.

Clinical signs

Strangles is characterised by the swelling of the lymph nodes (glands) below the horse's throat and profuse discharge from one or both nostrils.

First signs may include:
- raised temperature up to 40.5 °C (105 °F)
- watery discharge from one or both nostrils
- a soft, moist cough
- slight increase in respiratory rate
- dullness and lethargy.

As the disease progresses:

- the nasal discharge becomes thick and yellow (*Figure 14.5*)
- abscesses form in the lymph nodes under the throat and at the back of the pharynx. Developing abscesses are hot, hard and extremely painful: they may cause the horse to hold its head outstretched. Breathing is occasionally obstructed
- swallowing is painful, leading to depressed appetite and loss of condition
- over the next few days the abscesses increase in size and become softer (point). They eventually burst to release large amounts of pus. This occurs approximately 10–14 days after the start of the disease.

The pain is then relieved and the horse starts to recover (*Figure 14.6*).

When to call the vet

If you suspect strangles infection, contact your vet immediately. Early diagnosis and prompt action reduces the risk of a large outbreak occurring.

Diagnosis

Diagnosis is made on the clinical signs. It is confirmed by isolation of *Streptococcus equi* from swabs taken from the nasopharynx or burst abscesses.

Treatment

Careful nursing is essential.

Isolation

The horse should be isolated in a well-

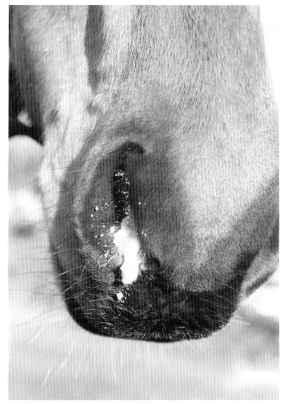

Figure 14.5   *Thick nasal discharge characteristic of strangles infection*

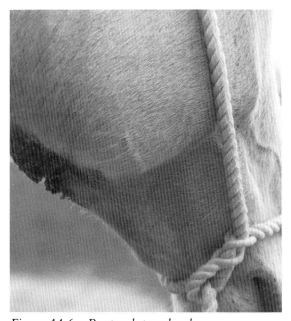

Figure 14.6   *Ruptured strangles abscess*

ventilated loose box. Dust levels must be kept to a minimum.

Feeding

- Offer soft, palatable mashes and hand-cut grass while swallowing is difficult.
- Soak the hay.

Water

- Affected horses often play with the water. They want to drink but are discouraged by discomfort when swallowing.
- As the head is lowered, large amounts of pus may be released into and around the bucket.

  The water should therefore be changed frequently and the buckets kept clean to encourage drinking.

Grazing

The horse can be turned out to graze provided it is isolated in a paddock well away from other horses.

N.B. This will contaminate the field for at least four weeks.

Abscesses

- Warm poultices or hot fomentations may be used to speed up maturation and rupture of the abscesses.
- Ruptured abscesses and those which the vet has lanced should be flushed out twice daily with a dilute solution of hydrogen peroxide.
- Nasal discharge should be wiped away with cotton wool and warm water as often as necessary.

Medication

Anti-inflammatory drugs, e.g. flunixin meglumine or phenylbutazone may be given early in the course of the disease. These lower the horse's temperature and reduce the pain and soft tissue swelling associated with the abscesses.

The use of antibiotics

In general, antibiotics are not used once the abscesses are forming. Antibiotics given at this stage can delay the maturation and rupture of the abscesses and so prolong the course of the disease.

Where factors such as the age of the horse and the severity of the condition give cause for concern, however, the vet may decide that antibiotics are necessary. Horses in an affected yard may therefore have different treatments.

When strangles is spreading through a group of horses, antibiotics can play an important role. In-contact horses often show a temperature rise before the onset of any other symptoms. A course of penicillin given at this stage may prevent the disease developing.

Antibiotics are sometimes given once the abscesses have ruptured in order to speed up elimination of the bacteria.

Inhalation of steam and medication

Inhalation of steam and vapours can provide considerable relief to a horse that is very congested or has a thick nasal discharge.

A few drops of oil of turpentine or eucalyptus oil are added to a bucket containing 0.5–1 litre of boiling water. The bucket is placed in a sack which is then held over the horse's nostrils.

The steaming is done twice a day for 5–10

minutes. Care should be taken not to restrict the horse's breathing in any way.

Alternatively, the oil can be dropped onto a piece of sponge or cotton wool inside a nosebag or muzzle. The nasal discharge runs out more freely after these procedures.

Owners' responsibilities

As soon as the disease is diagnosed, inform the owner(s) of any in-contact horses so they can check temperatures twice daily and be prepared to take immediate action.

Prevention and control

Bacteria are released into the environment when the horse coughs, and in the discharges.

As the disease is acquired by inhalation and ingestion of the bacteria, isolation and hygiene are of paramount importance.

Hygiene measures

- Isolate all affected horses.
- Where possible a separate groom should nurse the sick animals. Protective clothing such as overalls, boots, disposable gloves and a hat or scarf should be worn to prevent the spread of infection.
- Keep a bucket of disinfectant and brush outside each stable for cleaning boots when leaving the box.
- Use separate feed and water buckets.
- Burn all bedding, discharges and swabs from bathing the nostrils.
- Clean and disinfect rugs, headcollars and the stable once the horse has recovered.
- Do not turn affected horses out into paddocks shared with healthy animals as bacteria from the nasal discharge will remain infective for at least a month.

Hygiene measures should be continued for a month after the abscesses have ruptured as *Streptococcus equi* may still be shed by the horse. This causes further contamination of pastures, troughs, stables and equipment.

Points to remember

- The incubation period is 3–8 days.
- The whole yard must be treated as an isolation zone until four weeks after the last abscess has healed.
- No horses should go to public events such as shows, lessons or to visit other yards.
- No horses from outside should be allowed into the yard.

Return to work

The horse should be rested for at least 10 days after the abscesses have healed. Walking exercise may then be started.

Vaccination

There is no vaccine available in Britain.

Possible complications

Most cases of strangles recover with careful nursing.

Occasionally, the infection spreads to lymph nodes in other parts of the body and this is known as 'bastard strangles'.

When these abscesses are in superficial sites on the body, they burst without complications.

- In rare cases the swollen glands cause life-threatening respiratory obstruction. A temporary tracheotomy is necessary to relieve the airway.

- Drainage of abscesses into the trachea (windpipe) can cause pneumonia.
- Rupture of abscesses into the abdominal cavity can cause peritonitis and death.
- *Purpura haemorrhagica* may follow streptococcal infection in the horse.

Purpura Haemorrhagica

Purpura haemorrhagica is included in this section as it occasionally develops as a sequel to strangles and other streptococcal infections. It occurs 1–3 weeks after the horse appears to have recovered from the original infection.

Causes

It is an allergic reaction to the breakdown products of the bacteria (antigens), which circulate in the horse's bloodstream. The body produces antibodies to combine with and neutralise the antigen.

Instead of being filtered out by the lymph nodes, these antigen-antibody complexes continue to circulate and cause damage to the lining of blood vessels, allowing blood to escape into the tissues.

Clinical signs

Some or all of the following symptoms may be seen:
- oedema (swelling) of the nostrils, eyes and lips
- oedema of one or more limbs, which become very swollen (*Figure 14.7*)

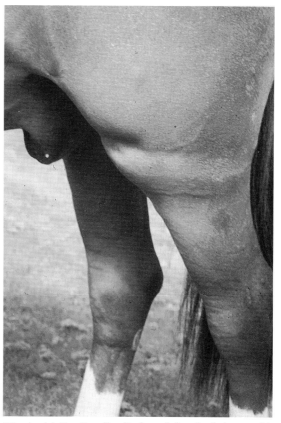

Figure 14.7 *Swollen limbs and sheath of a horse with purpura haemorrhagica*

- soft swellings anywhere on the body, especially the ventral abdomen
- bloodstained fluid (serum) may ooze through the skin
- stiffness and reluctance to move
- small haemorrhages on the lips and gums
- respiratory distress and swallowing difficulties due to fluid accumulation in the lungs and oedema of the larynx
- colic and bloodstained diarrhoea
- anaemia.

Treatment

This depends on which of the above symptoms are present. It may include the following drugs:

- antibiotics to kill the streptococci
- corticosteroids
- analgesic and anti-inflammatory drugs
- antihistamines
- diuretics.

In addition:
- vitamin K and calcium may help
- tracheotomy, blood transfusion and skin grafting are sometimes necessary.

Nursing

Good nursing is vital. The horse should be kept in a well-ventilated box with a clean comfortable bed.

Gentle exercise in hand helps decrease the swelling. The lower limbs should be covered with a tubular bandage to prevent bedding sticking to the exudate.

Prognosis

Even with the very best of care, only 50 per cent of affected horses will recover.

Pneumonia

Pneumonia is a bacterial infection of the lungs which is most commonly seen in foals. It rarely occurs in adult horses.

Causes

It can be caused by several types of bacteria which are either inhaled or enter the body of a newborn foal through the navel. These bac-

teria result in the formation of localised abscesses or inflammation of large areas of the lungs. Pneumonia can develop following:
- viral infection
- inhalation of food or liquid, e.g. from careless drenching or in any condition where the horse has swallowing difficulties
- stress, e.g. long journeys or insufficient rest after an upper respiratory tract infection.

Clinical signs

These may include:
- fever, 39–41 °C (103–106 °F)
- fast, shallow breathing
- coughing
- abnormal lung sounds
- mucopurulent nasal discharge (not always present)
- depression
- loss of appetite and condition.

When to call the vet

If you suspect your horse or foal has pneumonia, call the vet immediately.

Diagnosis

Diagnosis is made on the clinical signs.

The following procedures may also be used:
- blood samples
- tracheal wash
- radiography
- ultrasound scanning.

Treatment

Treatment depends on the severity of the

condition. It can include:
- a long course of antibiotics (usually 4–6 weeks)
- mucolytic and bronchodilator drugs
- non-steroidal anti-inflammatory drugs to reduce the fever and pain
- oxygen administered via a face mask
- intravenous fluids.

Nursing

The horse must be nursed in a well-ventilated box with a clean, deep bed. Where necessary, rugs should be used to keep the animal warm.

Offer soft, palatable food and ensure that clean drinking water is available.

Prognosis

The prognosis is guarded.

Lungworm

The donkey is the natural host of the lungworm, *Dictyocaulus arnfieldi*, but horses may also become infected.

Donkeys can have large numbers of these worms without showing any symptoms, whereas horses are more likely to develop clinical signs.

Clinical signs

Where symptoms are observed, they include:
- a chronic cough, especially during exercise
- increased respiratory rate.

Life-cycle

Adult worms and larvae live in the bronchi of infected donkeys. The eggs which the adults lay are coughed up and swallowed. They pass through the donkey's gut and reach the pasture in the faeces.

In the warm summer months, the larvae hatch quickly. If eaten by a horse or donkey, they burrow through the intestinal wall and pass to the lungs via the bloodstream or lymph vessels.

In a donkey, the larvae mature into adult worms and the cycle is repeated.

With many horses, however, the larvae in the lungs do not develop into adult worms and no eggs are produced.

Diagnosis

A diagnosis of lungworm in the horse is made on:
- clinical signs
- history of contact with a donkey
- tracheal wash
- faecal examination (usually negative but a few infected horses pass lungworm eggs)
- response to anthelmintic treatment.

The faeces of other horses and any donkeys sharing the field can also be tested.

Treatment

Immediate

Dose with a suitable anthelmintic, e.g. ivermectin. All the horses and donkeys in the field should be treated at the same time.

Long term

Infective larvae may survive on the pasture

for several months (even during the winter). Horses remaining in the field should be dosed at monthly intervals with ivermectin, fenbendazole or mebendazole at the recommended dose rate.

Prevention

Do not allow donkeys and horses to graze together.

N.B. Large numbers of *Parascaris equorum* (roundworm) in young animals can also cause respiratory symptoms.

Chronic Obstructive Pulmonary Disease (COPD)

COPD is an allergic condition which affects many horses.

Causes

It is caused by the horse being exposed to fungal spores and stable dust. The horse becomes hypersensitive to inhaled spores and experiences an asthma-type reaction.

Most particles of stable dust are filtered out as air passes through the nostrils and complex nasal passages. However, the spores of some moulds, e.g. *Aspergillus fumigatus* and the actinomycete *Faenia rectivirgula* (old name: *Micropolyspora faeni*) are small enough to reach the bronchioles where they cause inflammation.

This leads to increased production of mucus and spasm of smooth muscle in the airway walls. Both cause a reduction in airway diameter.

Clinical signs

The disease usually develops over a period of time. Affected horses do not have a temperature and they appear well in themselves. However, COPD causes reduced exercise tolerance. The first symptoms include:
• increased respiratory rate
• increased expiratory effort; the abdominal muscles are used to force the air from the lungs. This results in a marked and characteristic biphasic expiratory movement
• an occasional cough, usually at the start of exercise
• milky white nasal discharge, especially first thing in the morning and after exercise.

As the condition progresses:
• breathing out requires even more effort and there is considerable movement of the abdominal muscles; this is known as heaving
• the nasal discharge may become thick and yellow
• coughing may persist throughout exercise
• the horse may begin to cough at rest in the stable
• lumps of mucus are sometimes coughed up.

Once a horse has become sensitised, it may suffer acute attacks of the disease and develop severe respiratory difficulties in a short period of time. The animal breathes with flared nostrils and heaving flanks and has spells of continuous coughing.

When to call the vet

Call the vet at the first sign of the disease. Early diagnosis and treatment often prevent it from developing into a serious problem.

Diagnosis

Diagnosis is made on the clinical signs.

In the early stages, no abnormal lung sounds can be heard with the stethoscope. Severe cases have a wide range of abnormal lung sounds.

When the upper respiratory tract is examined with an endoscope, a stream of mucopus may be observed in the trachea (*Figure 14.8*).

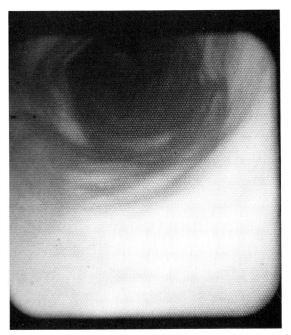

Figure 14.8 *Mucopus in the trachea*

Treatment and prevention

The key to both treatment and prevention of the disease is good stable management and stable design.

Turning out

All horses should have plenty of fresh air with minimal exposure to dust and fungal spores. Wherever possible, they should be turned out for a few hours each day.

The first step in the treatment of horses with COPD is to turn them out (night and day) for a period of at least three weeks.

When a clipped horse suffers an acute attack of the disease, it must be kept warm and dry using suitable rugs.

The field should be well away from the hay store.

Stable design

In mild cases, changes in stable management and modification of stable design may be all that is required to control the symptoms.

Good ventilation is essential for the horse's health. Many modern boxes have low roofs and insufficient air vents to achieve the minimum acceptable ventilation rate of six complete air changes per hour.

The ventilation of most boxes can be improved with relatively little expense. These improvements could include:

- additional air inlets and outlets. To avoid draughts at horse level, air inlets should be positioned at the same height as the eaves. Ideally, each stable should have an outlet in the roof
- top doors should always be left open. In extremely cold weather, put an extra rug on the horse
- side walls of the stable should reach the roof, ensuring that each horse has a separate air space. Dust free management procedures will be of less value if a horse sharing the same air space has dry hay and straw.

If you need advice on stable design, consult your vet.

Bedding

Straw is not ideal as it supports greater levels of fungal growth than a well managed peat, woodshavings or paper bed.

Wood shavings and paper beds need to be kept clean, or they also become contaminated by mould.

Deep litter is not recommended. In addition to fungal growth, high levels of noxious gases such as ammonia and hydrogen sulphide may be produced. These are irritant to the respiratory tract.

Mucking out

It is essential that *all* the bed is removed and replaced at regular intervals. Wood shavings that look clean can have high levels of fungal growth after several months in a stable.

Ledges and window sills must be regularly dusted.

During normal mucking out, the number of fungal spores in the atmosphere increases three- to six-fold. Many remain airborne for several hours. It therefore makes sense to muck out as soon as the horse is turned out so the spores have a chance to settle before the horse is brought in again.

The muck heap

The muck heap should be sited as far from the stables as possible and preferably downwind.

Diet

Concentrates

Molassed mixes and cubes are suitable as they are dust free. There is little chance of fungal contamination provided they are fresh.

Other concentrates should be moistened before feeding.

Forage

Where possible, hay should be excluded from the diet altogether. Grass and vacuum-packed forage, e.g. Horsehage are suitable alternatives. If hay is fed, it must be of excellent quality and well soaked (see below).

Buying hay

Always buy the best quality that is available, it is worth the additional cost. Examine the hay closely and ask to see an open bale. It should have a fresh, sweet smell and no visible mould or dust.

Storing hay

Hay should be stored in a separate building from the horse because millions of invisible fungal spores are released into the atmosphere when haynets are filled. This happens even with top quality hay.

In order to minimise fungal growth and wastage of the lower bales, they should be raised from the floor on wooden pallets.

Soaking hay

When a horse pulls dry hay from a haynet, large numbers of fungal spores become airborne and are inhaled.

Soaking the hay in a trough or large plastic dustbin for several hours significantly reduces the number of inhaled spores.

Only soak the amount that the horse will eat overnight, as it quickly becomes unpalatable. Any left over should be discarded.

Position the haynet so that there is minimal mixing with the bedding and dropped hay can be swept up and removed.

Vacuum-packed forage

Vacuum-packed forage has been developed

specifically for the horse as an alternative to hay. It is dust free.

Grass is cut and allowed to wilt before being baled and compressed. The bales are sealed in bags to exclude air and a mild fermentation process begins. Under these conditions, mould growth is inhibited and the feed will keep for up to 18 months.

Vacuum-packed forage has a higher nutritional value than most hay (it is also more expensive). It should be introduced to the diet over a period of 2–3 weeks and concentrates may need to be reduced.

Opened packs should be used within five days. If the bag is damaged when delivered it should be returned to the suppliers. Where a bag is accidentally punctured in the yard, it should be fed immediately.

A feeding guide can be obtained from the manufacturers. Haynets with small holes slow down the horse's intake of this forage.

Exercise

Mildly affected horses benefit from exercise. It helps to mobilise the mucus and keeps the respiratory system toned up. During a bout of coughing, the horse should be allowed to walk.

Horses with moderate to severe breathing difficulties should not be worked.

Medication

Medication alone is not the answer. However, when combined with dust-free management, the following drugs aid recovery.

Bronchodilators

These stop the spasm of smooth muscle in the airway walls.

Mucolytics

Mucolytic drugs reduce the viscosity of the mucus and help to mobilise it from the lower airways.

Antibiotics

These may be used if the discharge is mucopurulent and secondary infection is suspected.

Corticosteroids

Corticosteroids are sometimes used in acute cases. They reduce inflammation but cannot be used in the long term because of side effects.

Sodium cromoglycate

Sodium cromoglycate may prevent further attacks once the horse has been desensitised and is clinically normal. Fine droplets of the drug are inhaled using a face mask and a nebuliser. Four days of treatment gives 20 days of protection.

Transport

When travelling, horses are often exposed to high spore levels. Straw and shavings in lorries and trailers quickly become musty and mixed up with hay. The best solution is to use rubber matting and avoid feeding hay inside the vehicle.

Pasture Associated Pulmonary Disease (PAPD)

A number of horses develop the symptoms

of COPD while out at grass, with no exposure to hay. The condition is known as pasture associated pulmonary disease (PAPD).

Causes

These horses are thought to be allergic to a variety of pollens. Oilseed rape is currently suspected as being one cause of the condition.

Management and treatment

Management of these animals is very difficult; their environment should be kept as dust free as possible.

Medication may alleviate the symptoms until the pollen count has subsided.

Some animals show an immediate improvement when moved to another location.

Laryngeal Hemiplegia

Laryngeal hemiplegia (whistling and roaring) is a condition in which affected horses make a characteristic whistling or roaring sound due to obstruction of the airway.

Structure and function of the larynx

The larynx is situated in the horse's throat at the top of the trachea (windpipe). It is made up of several cartilages and ligaments, joined in such a way that the larynx can open and close.

The opening and closing of the larynx is controlled by several small muscles. Most of these are innervated by the right and left recurrent laryngeal nerves.

Normal movements of the larynx

When the horse swallows, the larynx closes to prevent inhalation of food.

During strenuous exercise, the larynx opens fully to allow maximum air flow to the lungs (*Figure 14.9*).

During resting respiration, the larynx is in an intermediate position. It opens a little wider during inspiration and narrows during expiration. The opening of the larynx is symmetrical and the movement is smooth and equal on both sides.

Laryngeal hemiplegia

For reasons that are not fully understood, the left recurrent laryngeal nerve degenerates in some horses. The muscles supplied by the damaged nerve waste away and the left side of the larynx is no longer capable of the normal range of movement.

During fast exercise, the flow of air is obstructed. This is due to incomplete opening of the left side of the larynx (*Figure 14.10*).

Clinical signs

The condition most commonly occurs in horses over 16 h.h. It is usually apparent by the time the horse is six years old.

- The horse makes an abnormal noise when it *breathes in* at canter and gallop. This is due to turbulence in the airstream as the air passes through the obstructed laryngeal opening. It may be a high pitched whistle or harsh roaring sound. In severe cases it can be heard at trot.

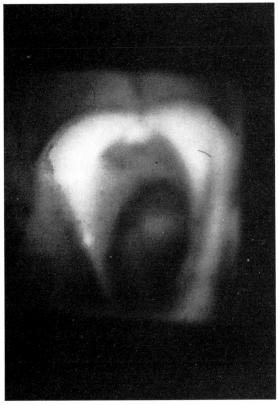

Figure 14.9   *Endoscopic view of a normal larynx following exercise*

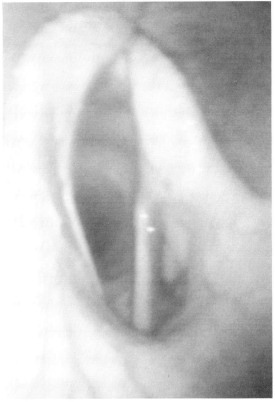

Figure 14.10   *Laryngeal hemiplegia: note the asymmetry of the laryngeal opening*

The noise should not be confused with normal expiratory (breathing out) sounds such as high blowing which is caused by air turbulence at the nostrils.

It is relatively easy to distinguish inspiratory and expiratory sounds. At canter and gallop, the horse's respiratory cycle is related to its stride. The horse exhales as the forelegs touch the ground.

- The horse may show reduced performance at exercise.
- The horse's voice may change.
- As the muscles on the left side of the larynx atrophy (waste away), parts of the laryngeal cartilages become more prominent and may be palpated through the skin.

Diagnosis

Diagnosis is made on the clinical findings:
- abnormal inspiratory noise
- laryngeal palpation
- endoscopy.

Endoscopic findings

The larynx is examined at rest and immediately after strenuous exercise. Endoscopy is necessary to assess the degree of paralysis as well as to confirm the diagnosis. (Laryngeal hemiplegia is not the only cause of inspiratory noise.)

When a horse has complete laryngeal hemiplegia, there is no active movement of the left side of the larynx. The opening appears markedly asymmetrical. Even after strenuous exercise, the left side does not move from the resting position.

More commonly, the larynx is only partially paralysed. The observed range of movement is either reduced or exaggerated and jerky.

Treatment

There is no cure for the disease. The nerve and muscle activity will never return.

There are three options the vet will consider.

1) *No treatment*. Many horses perform satisfactorily despite making a noise.

2) *Hobday operation*. This is the traditional treatment for partial paralysis.

A small pocket of tissue (the lateral ventricle) is removed from the left side of the larynx. This may reduce the turbulence of air as it passes through the larynx so the horse makes less noise.

3) *Abductor muscle prosthesis*. In cases of complete or severe paralysis, the muscle that opens the left side of the larynx is replaced with a prosthesis. A band of material is used to tie the left side of the larynx in the open position.

The operation is usually successful in relieving obstruction of the airway, but it is not without complications. With the larynx held permanently open, food sometimes enters the trachea during swallowing. For a small number of horses, this is a serious problem and the horse is left with a persistent cough.

15 Skin Problems

The Structure and Function of Skin

Skin is the outer, protective covering of the body (*Figure 15.1*). It has a complex structure which allows it to perform many important functions.

For descriptive purposes, skin can be divided into two layers: the outer epidermis and the inner dermis.

Epidermis

The *epidermis* is composed of several layers of cells. The cells of the deepest layer divide all

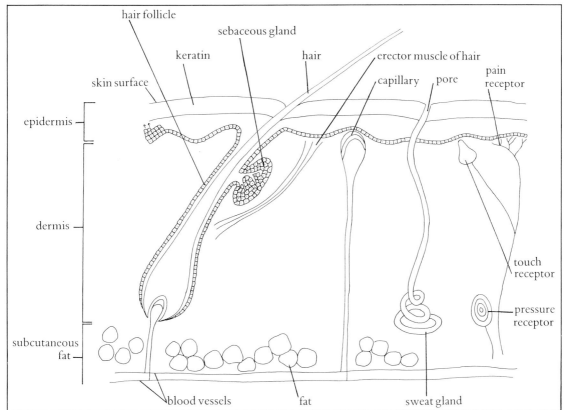

Figure 15.1   *Diagrammatic section through the skin*

the time and are pushed up towards the surface to replace those that continually wear away or flake off. As the cells are pushed up to the surface, they die and become transformed into a tough protein material called *keratin*.

Keratin is virtually waterproof. It prevents water evaporating from the living tissues underneath. It also stops the skin absorbing water.

Another function of the tough epidermis is to act as a barrier, preventing bacteria from entering the body.

Dermis

The underlying *dermis* consists of loose connective tissue, containing strong collagen fibres and elastic fibres. These give the skin its properties of strength and elasticity so it keeps its shape and is resistant to tearing.

Within the dermis are *hair follicles*, *sweat* and *sebaceous glands*, *blood vessels* and *nerve endings*.

Most of the horse's body is covered with *hair*. This protects the skin from injury and keeps the horse warm. Each hair grows from a hair follicle. Attached to this is a small band of muscle. When the weather is cold, the muscle contracts, causing the hair to stand up. The extra air trapped between the hairs is a poor conductor of heat and acts as a warm insulating layer.

Opening into the hair follicle is a sebaceous gland which produces an oily substance. This coats the hair, preventing it from becoming dry and brittle. It also helps to waterproof the skin surface.

Sweat glands consist of long coiled tubes which open onto the skin surface. When sweat evaporates, the skin surface is cooled.

The skin's blood vessels bring oxygen and nutrients to the living cells. They also play an important role in temperature regulation. On a very cold day, the vessels near the skin surface constrict. The reduced blood flow lessens the heat lost to the atmosphere by

radiation. Conversely, when a horse is warm, these vessels dilate and more heat is lost from the body.

Skin has numerous nerve endings. These supply the brain with continuous information about touch, pressure, cold, heat and pain. Perception of these sensations allows the horse to move away from unfavourable stimuli.

In addition to these protective functions, the skin synthesises vitamin D in sunlight.

As the largest and most exposed organ in the body, the skin is subject to a variety of ailments.

Ringworm

Ringworm is a fungal infection of the skin. It is caused by *Trichophyton spp.* and *Microsporum spp.*

Clinical signs

The lesions are very variable in appearance (*Figures 15.2–15.6*). In the early stages, tufts of hair may stand up from the rest of the coat. Affected areas vary in size from a couple of millimetres up to 4 or 5 cm. They are often round but can be any shape.

The tufts of hair then fall out. The hairs are stuck together by a crust of exudate. The skin beneath the scabs may exude serum. When this dries up, the lesions become dry and scaly. Hair regrows approximately four weeks later.

In other cases, the hair breaks off and the lesions are dry and scaly from the start. The typically circular patches enlarge as the fungus spreads outwards from the edge of the lesion (*Figure 15.4*).

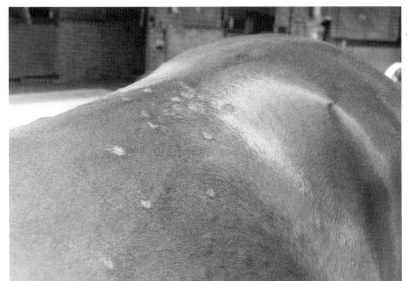

Figure 15.2 *Multiple patches of ringworm on a horse's back*

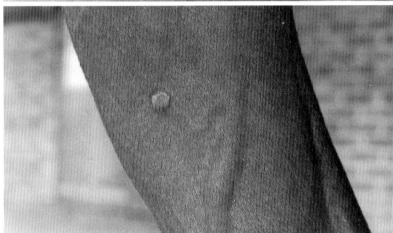

Figure 15.3 *Single ringworm lesion on a hind leg*

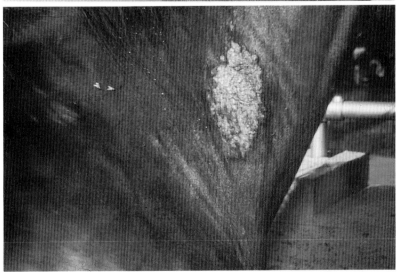

Figure 15.4 *Dry, scaly patch of ringworm on a horse's neck*

Figure 15.5   *Ringworm lesions are very variable in appearance*

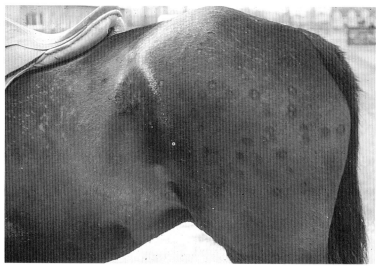

Figure 15.6   *Ringworm lesions can be widespread over the horse's body*

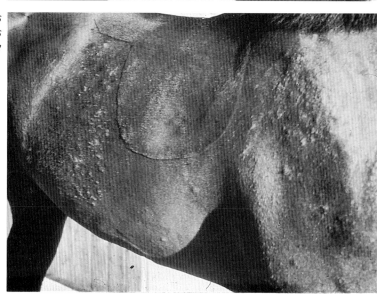

Common sites

The lesions can occur anywhere on the body, but the most commonly affected areas are the head, neck, girth and saddle regions.

Diagnosis

Diagnosis is made on:
• clinical examination

• history, e.g. are any other horses affected? Ringworm is very contagious so outbreaks often occur
• microscopic examination of hair and crusts of exudate for the presence of the fungus
• culture of the fungus; results take up to 10 days.

Treatment

The disease can be spread by direct contact,

so infected horses should be isolated wherever possible.

Systemic and topical treatments are normally recommended, together with a number of hygiene measures. Where a horse has just one or two discrete lesions, topical treatment combined with hygiene measures may suffice.

Topical treatment

There is a wide variety of drugs on the market for spraying or sponging onto the horse.

The treatment is usually applied on two or three occasions at three day intervals. Resistant lesions are treated again two weeks later.

Strong iodine is very effective for killing ringworm. However, it may blister thin-skinned horses and should never be used near the eyes.

Systemic treatment

Griseofulvin is an antifungal antibiotic given by mouth. Following absorption from the gut, the drug is incorporated into the skin and hair structure. This helps the skin resist fungal attack. A course of treatment lasts for a minimum of seven days.

N.B. *Griseofulvin must not be given to pregnant mares.* It is teratogenic, i.e. it can cause abnormalities in the developing foal.

Control

The fungi produce a large number of spores which are released into the environment. These remain infective for months or years. The following measures help reduce the spread of spores and therefore reduce environmental contamination.

As soon as ringworm is diagnosed:
1) Begin topical and systemic medication.
2) Stop grooming the horse as this spreads the infectious spores all over the coat.
3) Soak brushes, rugs, tack, etc. in a fungicidal solution. Horse clothing and grooming kit must not be shared between horses.
4) If the horse is rugged up, use a cotton summer sheet next to the skin as this is easy to wash. It should be soaked in a fungicide at least twice a week. Some saddlers will treat New Zealand and jute rugs to kill ringworm spores.
5) Never clip a horse with ringworm. It contaminates the clippers and spreads the infection.
6) If the girth and saddle areas are affected, do not ride the horse. Remember to treat your riding boots. In the recovery stages, washable numnahs and girth sleeves should be used.

Handling infected horses

The spores can be passed from one horse to another on clothing and hands.

Therefore:
- if one person has to handle several horses, the infected animals should be seen to last
- wear an overall to protect your clothes from contamination
- always wash your hands after handling an infected horse. *Remember, ringworm infects humans as well as horses.*

Treating the stable

Wherever possible, the stable should be treated. This entails removing and burning all of the bedding. Any faecal material or bedding which remains stuck to the walls must be scrubbed off. The walls, doors, etc. should then be washed with a fungicide. Wood should be creosoted.

Competing and travelling

Do not compete or travel to shows while the lesions are active. Lorries and trailers will become contaminated and the disease will be spread.

Daily inspection

Check daily for lesions developing on other horses in the yard. The incubation period is 7–14 days.

Other information

The disease is self-limiting and if left untreated will normally resolve in 6–12 weeks. The horse is usually resistant to reinfection for several months after recovery.

Sweet Itch

Sweet itch is an allergic skin condition causing horses and ponies to rub their manes and tails. It is more common in ponies than horses.

Causes

Affected animals are hypersensitive to a protein in the saliva of the biting *Culicoides* midge.

Clinical signs

The condition varies in severity from occa-

sional rubbing with some broken mane and tail hairs to almost complete loss of the mane and tail.

The symptoms are most obvious from April until November, but occasionally remain throughout the winter.

- Affected ponies rub their manes and tails against trees, fences and stables (*Figures 15.7 and 15.8*).
- Some animals become scurfy and itchy along the whole length of their backs.
- Persistent rubbing can cause bald patches and open sores on the head, neck, withers, shoulders, rump and dock.
- Secondary bacterial infection can develop.
- With time, the repeated trauma causes thickening and ridging of the skin at the base of the mane (*Figure 15.7*).

Treatment and prevention

With ponies that suffer every year, you should aim to *prevent* the symptoms by careful management, rather than waiting for them to develop.

The two most important considerations are:
- reducing exposure to the midges
- relieving the irritation.

Management

The midges breed in standing water and damp, rotting vegetation. They feed primarily at dawn and dusk. Therefore, wherever possible:
- move affected ponies out of marshy fields and away from rivers and lakes
- stable them between 4 p.m. and 8 a.m.
- screen the stable windows and half door with a very fine mesh to stop entry of the midges
- keep water barrels and stagnant troughs away from the stable
- use a summer sheet to protect the base of

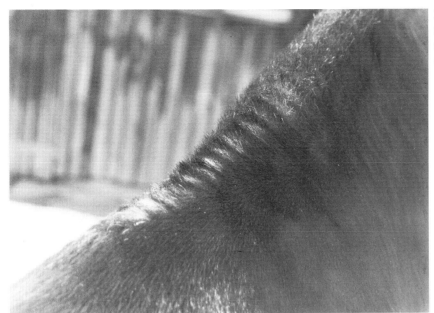

Figure 15.7 *Sweet itch: note the thickening and ridging of the skin at the base of the mane*

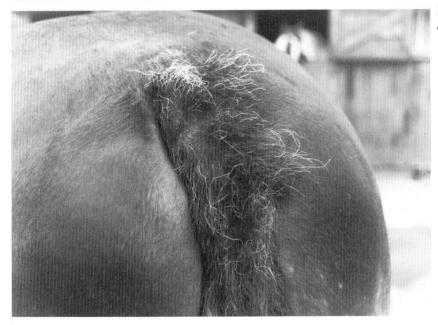

Figure 15.8 *Sweet itch: a badly-rubbed tail*

the mane and tail; complete neck and tail covers help a number of ponies
- some owners report an improvement with the inclusion of garlic in the diet
- access to a magnesium-rich mineral block is reported to cause a marked improvement in the condition of some affected animals.

Topical applications

- Fly repellent: use a fly repellent twice daily or a long-acting repellent every few days.
- Soothing lotions: there are many oily lotions on the market which make the pony less attractive to the midges and have a soothing effect, e.g. benzyl benzoate.

The lotion should be applied once or twice daily, according to the manufacturer's instructions.

It must be rubbed well into the skin of the dock and under the mane.

Parting the hair at intervals and using a water brush helps to ensure even distribution. Always wear rubber gloves and wash your hands afterwards.

- Shampoo: a shampoo with careful rinsing every 1–2 weeks helps to remove the scurf and scabs.
- A corticosteroid cream may be prescribed to soothe sore, inflamed areas.

Systemic treatment

Long-acting corticosteroid injections used to be given to reduce the irritation. However, the drug has many side-effects and may occasionally precipitate laminitis with rotation of the pedal bone in susceptible animals. For this reason, corticosteroids are no longer used as a routine treatment.

Prognosis

The prognosis is guarded.

The disease can be both debilitating and disfiguring. It prevents the animal being used for showing and the sores may limit riding in the summer.

Sweet itch is costly in time, effort and money. Not surprisingly, affected ponies may become bad-tempered and unreliable.

There are a few ponies for whom no treatment is effective. If every summer is a time of torment and misery, then euthanasia may have to be considered.

Other information

Many of these animals are sold during the winter months and the problem is passed on to another unsuspecting owner. Purchasers should always be warned about the condition as these ponies require special attention and should go to experienced homes with suitable facilities.

Breeding

Affected animals should not be used for breeding as the condition is hereditary.

Mud Fever

This common condition affects horses living or working in muddy conditions.

Causes

The constant wetting of the skin and irritation from the mud allows infection by the actinomycete *Dermatophilus congolensis*.

Clinical signs

These are as follows:

Sites of infection

The back of the pastern and the heels are most commonly affected (*Figures 15.9 and 15.10*). White legs are particularly susceptible. The infection may extend to the skin over the tendons, the inside of the thighs and the belly.

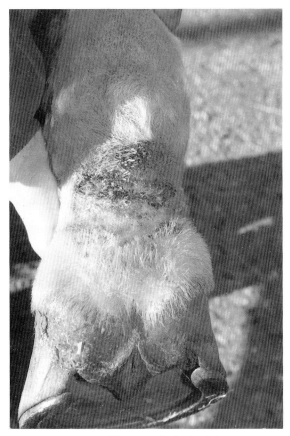

Figure 15.9   *Mud fever on the back of the pastern*

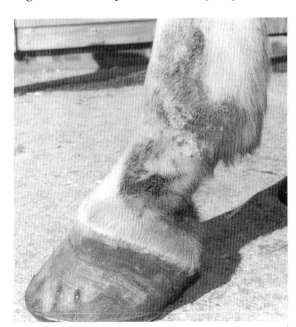

Figure 15.10   *Mud fever on the pastern and fetlock*

Mild cases

With mild cases there are a few small, scabby areas of skin. These require prompt attention or a more serious infection may develop.

Severe cases

In a severe case, larger areas of skin become inflamed. They exude serum which mats the hair in clumps. The skin is very sore. There may be considerable swelling of the lower limb and the horse is often lame.

Treatment

This will vary depending on the severity of the condition.

Mild cases

1) The first step in treating any case of mud fever is to remove the horse from the cause, i.e. the wet and the mud. If at all possible, stable the horse.
2) Clip hair from around the affected area using curved scissors.
3) Gently remove the scabs. This is necessary to allow the drugs to be brought into contact with the infecting organisms on the skin surface.
4) Apply a soothing antibiotic ointment, e.g. Dermobion, to the damaged skin twice daily.
   The corticosteroid in the ointment helps reduce the inflammation.
5) Stable bandages applied over clean Gamgee prevent bedding from sticking to the treated areas.
6) If you have an empty stable without any bedding, the horse can stand with no bandages for a few hours during the day.

7) Exercise may be continued, but avoid muddy areas – stick to roadwork and avoid the puddles!

Severe cases

With a severe case of mud fever the legs become very swollen and sore. They are frequently contaminated with mud and bedding material and secondary bacterial infection may develop. A course of antibiotics is usually prescribed to clear up the infection.

These horses *must* be stabled.

Although the aim is to dry up the infection, it is occasionally necessary to poultice the legs in the initial stages of treatment. The steps are:
1) Clip the hair away.
2) Gently wash off as much mud and debris as you can using warm water, cotton wool and a bactericidal soap, e.g. Hibiscrub or Pevidine.
3) Apply a warm poultice, e.g. Animalintex, which has been squeezed as dry as possible. This will draw out dirt and infection and the warmth will increase the blood supply to the damaged skin.
4) When the poultice is removed, gently wash off the sticky gel and remove as many of the scabs as possible.

   This is obviously very painful and, in some cases, it may be necessary to remove the scabs in stages. You may need to ask your vet to administer a sedative.
5) Dry the legs thoroughly and apply a soothing antibacterial ointment under a layer of Gamgee and a stable bandage. The bandages should not be tight and must extend from below the knee or hock to the coronary band.

   If the horse objects to its legs being touched, spread the ointment onto the Gamgee or a non-stick dressing rather than directly onto the leg.
6) Re-dress the legs once or twice daily. When the exudation stops, leave the horse

in a stable with no bedding and the legs unbandaged for a few hours.
7) Gentle exercise in hand helps to reduce the swelling.

Prevention

Be very vigilant and inspect your horse's legs carefully each day if it is prone to mud fever. Begin treatment at the first sign of infection.

Applying zinc and castor oil or liquid paraffin to the heels and pasterns before working in muddy conditions may reduce the incidence of the disease in susceptible horses. The legs must be clean and dry when these are applied.

When cleaning horses brought in from a muddy field, sponge or hose off the wet mud then dry the legs thoroughly. Alternatively, if the mud is nearly dry, you can apply stable bandages to speed drying and brush it off later. Avoid using a stiff brush on wet muddy skin.

Clip long hair from the legs of susceptible animals.

Rain Scald

Rain scald is a skin infection seen in horses and ponies at grass (*Figures 15.11–15.13*).

Causes

Prolonged or driving rain leads to excessive wetting of the skin. The actinomycete, *Dermatophilus congolensis* is able to penetrate the softened skin and cause an exudative dermatitis. This organism also causes mud fever and cracked heels.

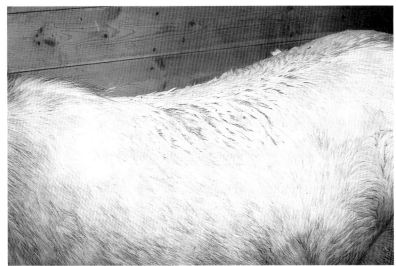

Figure 15.11   *Rain scald on a pony's back*

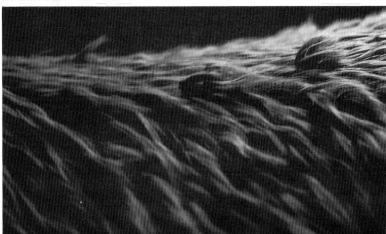

Figure 15.12   *Close up view of rain scald showing the matted clumps of hair*

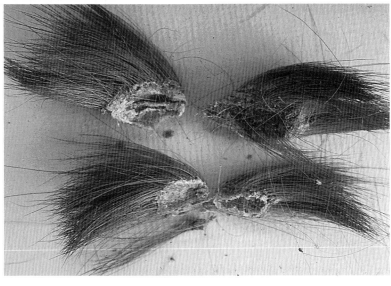

Figure 15.13   *The tufts of hair can be lifted off with a crust of exudate*

Clinical signs

- The most commonly affected areas are the back, loins, quarters and shoulders
- Large tufts of hair become matted together. These can be gently teased off together with a thick crust of exudate. The underlying skin may be dry and flaky or it may exude serum
- If secondary infection is present, a thick layer of pus is found under the scabs.

Treatment

Stable the horse until the lesions have healed. It is very difficult to clear the infection if the horse is still exposed to rain.

Gently tease off the scabs. Where these are small and widespread throughout the coat, a fine-toothed metal comb removes them very effectively.

If there is exudate under the large scabs, clean the skin with cotton wool and an anti-bacterial wash, e.g. Hibiscrub or Pevidine.

In severe cases veterinary advice should be sought because a course of antibiotics may be necessary.

The horse should remain stabled until the skin is dry and healthy. It can then be turned out wearing a New Zealand rug.

Prevention

- Provide shelter.
- Use a New Zealand rug.

Lice

There are two types of louse that live on horses. *Haematopinus asini*, the sucking louse, feeds on blood and tissue fluids. *Damalinia equi*, the biting louse, feeds on scurf and other debris on the skin surface.

Infestations usually occur in the winter months when the coat is long. Lice are visible to the naked eye. They are 1.5–3 mm long and grey in colour. The cream-coloured eggs (known as 'nits'), are usually found close to the roots of the mane and around the forelock.

These lice are host-specific and do not live on humans.

Clinical signs

Lice cause the skin to become very itchy. Infested horses rub and bite themselves, creating bald and sore patches (*Figure 15.14*). The coat becomes dull and scurfy.

Severely infested animals become restless and lose condition.

If left untreated, the skin eventually becomes thickened.

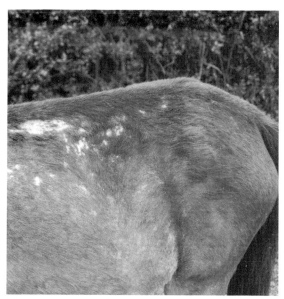

Figure 15.14 *Bald patches caused by rubbing and biting due to severe infestation of lice*

Treatment

Antiparasitic washes or louse powder should be applied. These preparations should be evenly distributed and well rubbed in. A second treatment two weeks later kills young lice that have hatched from the eggs since the first treatment.

Control

Lice spread from one animal to another by direct contact or via shared brushes, rugs, etc.

If one horse is affected, all the other horses in the field should be treated at the same time.

Warts and Tumours

There are several types of growth that affect the skin of horses and ponies. They are not usually painful but are a nuisance when they grow in inconvenient sites or spoil the horse's appearance. Some examples are described below.

Papilloma

Papillomas are small warts that are found in clusters on the lips and muzzle of young horses (*Figure 15.15*). They are occasionally seen on the ears and eyelids. They are unsightly, but rarely worry the animal.

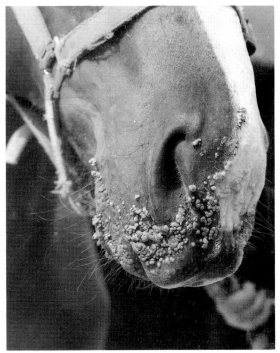

Figure 15.15 *Papillomas on the lips and muzzle of a young Thoroughbred*

Causes

Papillomas are caused by a virus and will disappear spontaneously.

Treatment

The only treatment required is cleaning of the skin if a papilloma is accidentally knocked and bleeds.

Melanoma

A melanoma is a tumour. It is found in horses

of all colours, but is most common in ageing greys (*Figure 15.16*).

Appearance

In hairless regions of the horse's skin, melanomas have a black, knobbly appearance. On the head, the growths are usually covered by hair.

Usual sites

Melanomas are usually located :
- on the underside of the dock
- around the anus
- the vulva
- the sheath
- the head.

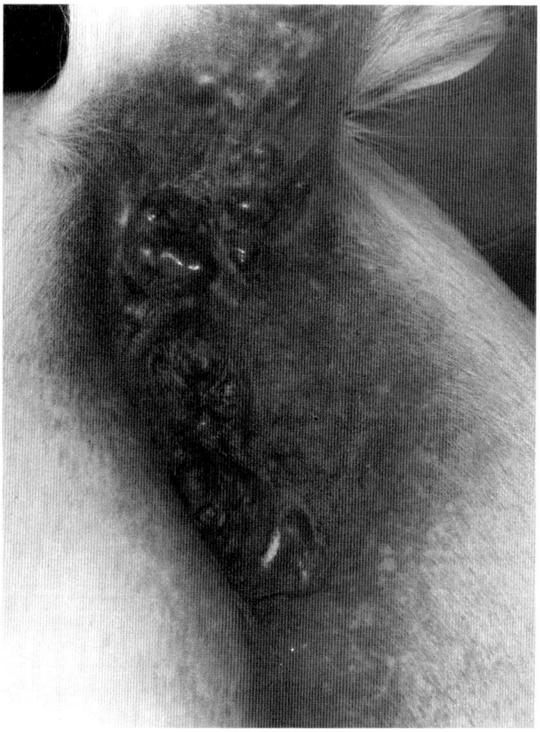

Treatment

Treatment is only required if the tumours ulcerate and become infected. This sometimes happens with large growths under the tail.

Melanomas are not routinely removed because they tend to develop in sites that are awkward for surgery and they often regrow.

Prognosis

Most elderly grey horses have at least one melanoma. They grow very slowly and rarely cause any problems.

Occasionally, melanomas spread rapidly throughout the body. In these cases, the prognosis is hopeless.

Figure 15.16   *Melanomas on an aged stallion*

Sarcoid

Sarcoids are the commonest skin tumour of the horse.

Appearance

Their appearance is variable. They may be:
- crusty and wart-like
- smooth and nodular
- flat, slightly bumpy areas of skin with hair loss, resembling ringworm in appearance.

Sarcoids may occur singly or in clusters. Their size varies from a few millimetres to several centimetres.

As they grow in size, sarcoids frequently ulcerate and become infected (*Figure 15.17*). Once this has occurred, they attract flies and do not heal.

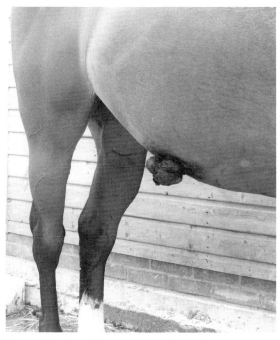

Figure 15.17   *A large ulcerated sarcoid*

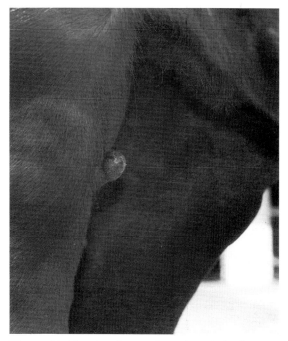

Figure 15.18   *Small sarcoid on a horse's thigh*

Common sites

They are normally found on:
- the inside of the thighs (*Figure 15.18*)
- on or around the sheath and udder
- behind the elbows and the girth area
- underneath the belly
- the head and neck.

Treatment

Sarcoids are notorious for recurring and developing at other sites, regardless of their management. However, early treatment gives the best results.

The options include:
- applying a tight elastic band around the base of the tumour
- surgical removal
- cryosurgery
- injection of BCG vaccine.

Your vet will decide on the most suitable approach. The decision will depend on the site, size and number of the tumours.

Each line of treatment has advantages and disadvantages; they are outlined below.

The elastic band

Method

This method is quick and simple, but only suitable for single tumours with a narrow base. A special instrument is used to place a thick rubber band around the neck of the tumour; this cuts off its blood supply.

Expected response

There is usually quite a lot of swelling and some discharge before the tumour drops off 2–3 weeks later.

Surgical removal

Method

This is performed under local or general anaesthesia. The tumours are removed together with a margin of healthy skin.

Wherever possible, the wound is closed with sutures. If the wound is too large to close, the area is left to heal on its own. In the meantime, it must be kept clean and dry.

The sutures are removed 10 days later. These wounds break down more often than other wounds; they must then heal by second intention (see Wound Healing, Chapter 2).

Cryosurgery

Method

This involves freezing the tumour to −25 °C and allowing it to thaw slowly. The freezing is then repeated. The procedure may be done under deep sedation with accessible sites, but often requires general anaesthesia. The advantage with this procedure is that it may stimulate the horse's immune system to reject further tumour growth.

Expected response

The tumour tissue dies and sloughs off over the next couple of weeks. There is a lot of discharge as the tissue dies. The area must be cleaned regularly and thoroughly.

Injection of BCG vaccine

Method

This method is useful for awkward sites, e.g. the eyelids, where surgical removal is inappropriate.

BCG vaccine is injected into the tumour. The horse's immune system recognises the vaccine as foreign and rejects it from the body.

Expected response

There is localised swelling, ulceration and pus accumulation around the injection site. The activated immune system may recognise the tumour as being foreign and reject it at the same time.

The treatment is repeated at 1–3 week intervals until regression occurs. It is successful in 50–60 per cent of cases.

The major drawback of this technique is the small risk of anaphylactic shock caused by injection of foreign protein.

Saddle Sores

These are sore patches of skin that develop under the saddle.

Causes

Saddle sores (*Figure 15.19*) are usually caused by poor stable management, e.g.:
• incorrectly fitted saddles
• unevenly stuffed saddles
• dirty saddles and numnahs
• overtight rollers with insufficient padding.

They can also be caused by bad riding.

Clinical signs

These include:
• patches of rubbed hair on the horse's back
• raised, thickened areas of skin
• tender areas, shown by resentment of grooming, saddling or mounting
• new patches of white hair.

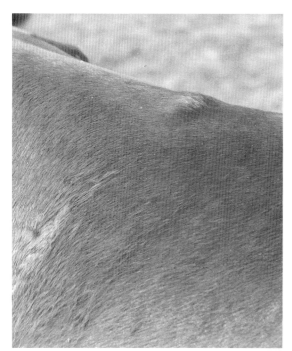

Figure 15.19 *Lump on a horse's back, caused by saddle pressure*

Points to look for when fitting a saddle

A well-fitted saddle distributes the weight of the rider evenly over a large area of the horse's back. It ensures that there is no pressure directly over the dorsal spinous processes.

Side view

From the side, the panel should fit snugly along the contours of the back. It should not extend as far back as the loins.

Withers

These should not be pinched or subjected to pressure. As a general guide, you should be able to fit three fingers between the withers and the pommel when the rider is mounted.

Gullet

This must be wide enough to prevent pinching of the spine.

Stuffing

This should be sufficient to allow daylight to be seen along the length of the gullet when the rider is mounted. The stuffing must be evenly distributed as lumps or ridges will make the back sore. Over-stuffing can make the panels too hard, causing pressure points.

Treatment

The damaged area must be protected from further trauma. Rest the horse or restrict exercise to lungeing without a saddle.

If the skin is broken, wash with warm water or sterile saline and cotton wool.

Dry the area and apply an antiseptic ointment or wound powder. Keep the area clean and dry until healing is complete.

The newly-healed skin can be hardened by regular applications of surgical spirit. It must then be protected by using a thick numnah or shock-absorbing gel pad.

Do not ride the horse until the wound has healed and the skin is no longer tender.

Prevention

Check the fitting of the saddle regularly.

The role of the saddler

If you are not sure whether a saddle fits

correctly ask an experienced saddler to come and advise you. Horses change shape as they mature and as they lose or gain weight. The saddle that fitted perfectly six months ago may well be causing problems now.

Rider problems

A rider who is out of balance or crooked will cause uneven pressure and increase the risk of saddle sores.

Numnahs

Numnahs cushion the horse's back from pressure and jarring. Some types, e.g. gel pads, have been developed to distribute pressure more evenly.

Cleanliness

- Groom the horse thoroughly before saddling.
- Wash numnahs regularly.
- Wash sweat from the saddle area.
- Keep the saddle clean and supple.

N.B. Care should be taken when washing horses and tack as some horses are allergic to biological detergents.

Sitfast

A sitfast is a core of dead skin in the saddle region. It is usually circular and approximately 1 cm in diameter.

Causes

A sitfast forms as a result of pressure from the saddle.

Treatment

It can sometimes be removed by poulticing but surgical removal may be necessary.

Girth Galls

A girth gall is a sore area that develops under the girth (*Figures 15.20 and 15.21*).

Causes

- A dirty girth with accumulated mud and sweat.
- Old or damaged girths.
- Loose girths rubbing the skin.
- Too tight a girth on a fat pony.
- Girthing over dirt.
- Unusually sensitive skin.

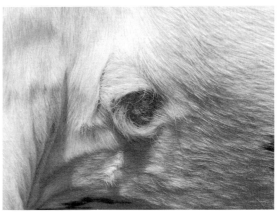

Figure 15.20   *A girth gall*

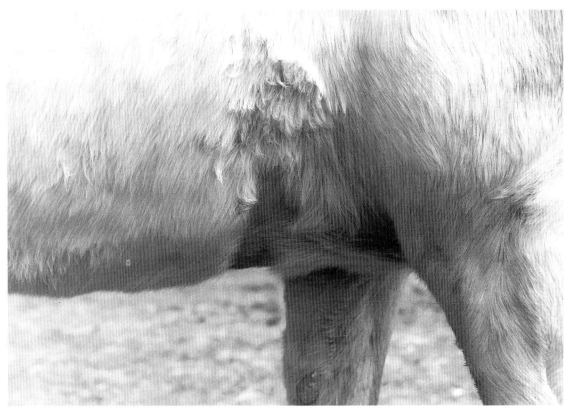

Figure 15.21   *Sore skin in the girth region*

Treatment

A girth gall should be managed in the same way as a saddle sore.

Exercise may be continued by lungeing without a saddle or roller.

Prevention

- Sensitive skin can be hardened by daily applications of surgical spirit.
- Use a washable girth sleeve or a tyre inner tube over the girth of susceptible animals. These can also be used in the recovery stages.
- Keep leather girths well oiled.
- Keep all girths clean and dry.

- Make sure the saddle and girth regions are free from mud before saddling up.

Urticaria (Nettle Rash)

Urticaria is an allergic reaction of the skin, sometimes known as 'nettle rash'.

Causes

There are a number of recognised causes of

urticaria. These include:
- components of the diet, e.g. barley
- fly bites
- nettles or other irritants
- drugs, e.g. some antibiotics.

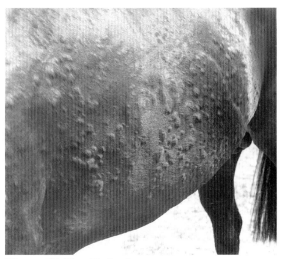

Figure 15.22   *Urticaria*

Clinical signs

The skin develops raised patches due to the accumulation of fluid in the dermis (*Figure 15.22*). The raised patches vary in size from 0.5 cm to the size of a saucer. They are painless when touched, but the skin may be itchy, causing the horse to rub and bite itself.

Serum sometimes oozes through the skin.

In severe cases the horse becomes distressed and shows colicky signs.

Common sites

The patches are irregularly distributed over the neck, the chest wall and the abdomen. The eyelids and muzzle sometimes swell.

When to call the vet

The lesions develop very quickly and will often disappear within a few hours without treatment. You should call the vet if:
- the horse is distressed
- the eyelids and muzzle are swollen
- serum is leaking through the skin
- there is no improvement after 24 hours
- the rash develops while the horse is being treated with drugs
- it interrupts a training programme.

Treatment

Treatment will depend on the severity of the condition.

Diet

A horse with urticaria should be given a light diet. Begin with a bran mash containing 100 g (4 oz) of Epsom salts – 50 g (2 oz) for a pony.

Avoid barley and high performance concentrates until the condition has resolved.

Medication

In severe cases, the vet may prescribe drugs to speed up recovery.

These may include:
- corticosteroids
- antihistamines
- antibiotics
- non-steroidal anti-inflammatory drugs.

Management

If the lesions are persistent, you should try to pinpoint the cause. The horse's management can then be adjusted to prevent it being exposed to the allergen.

Prevention

When a horse is known to have allergic reactions, commonsense preventive measures should be taken, e.g.:

- do not ride through stinging nettles
- cut down or spray nettles in the field
- apply fly repellent
- provide a shelter from flies
- use a summer sheet
- test new products on a small area of skin first
- use only proprietary horse shampoos
- avoid using biological detergents for rugs, numnahs and girths.

Photosensitisation

This is a condition where pink or lightly pigmented skin reacts abnormally to sunlight.

Causes

Photosensitisation occurs when a horse eats certain plants or has liver disease.

Some plants, e.g. St John's Wort and various clovers contain photodynamic agents which are absorbed by the horse's gut and reach the skin. Here they absorb energy from sunlight and this damages the surrounding cells.

Liver disease

Bacteria in the gut break down the chlorophyll in plants to a product called phylloerythrin. This is normally removed from the circulation by the liver and excreted in the bile.

With liver disease, excretion of bile is reduced and some phylloerythrin stays in the circulation. When it reaches the skin it can cause photosensitisation.

Clinical signs

- Non-pigmented areas of skin on the face and lower limbs are most commonly affected.
- The skin becomes swollen, inflamed and itchy.
- Serum exudes onto the skin surface.
- Secondary bacterial infection often develops.
- In severe cases, the skin dies and begins to slough.
- The affected areas are very sore.

Diagnosis

Diagnosis is made on the clinical signs.

Blood tests should be taken to check the liver function, and the field must be checked for any poisonous plants.

Treatment

This will include the following:

Stable management

The horse must be stabled until the condition has resolved.

A horse with a sore, cracked muzzle will find it easier to eat hay from the floor rather than pull it from a net. The hay should be well soaked to reduce dust levels.

Cleaning

Even when the skin is very sore it must be cleaned regularly. This should be done gently with lukewarm water, a bactericidal soap and cotton wool. After drying the area, apply an ointment containing antibiotic and a corticosteroid, e.g. Dermobion. This will reduce the inflammation and help protect against secondary bacterial infection.

Systemic treatment

The vet may administer antibiotics, antihistamines or corticosteroids. The treatment depends on the severity of the reaction and the cause of the condition.

Clinical signs

It most commonly affects the muzzle. The skin becomes very pink and develops scabby patches which sometimes become infected.

Treatment

Keep the horse out of bright sunlight and apply a soothing antibacterial ointment.

Prevention

Sunburn can be prevented by using topical sunscreens or stabling susceptible animals on hot, sunny days.

Sunburn

Photosensitisation is not the same as sunburn (*Figure 15.23*) which is a normal reaction of non-pigmented (pink) skin to sunlight.

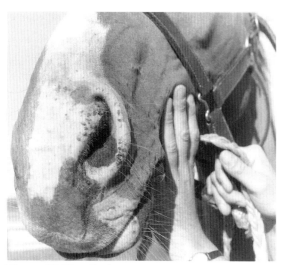

Figure 15.23   *Sunburn*

Vitiligo

Vitiligo is the name given to a condition where patches of skin lose their pigmentation and become pink in colour.

Causes and clinical signs

It can be caused by badly fitting tack or harness. The pigment cells are destroyed and pink areas develop. It occurs at the corners of the mouth and the side of the dock when rubber guards are used on the bit and crupper.

The condition can also arise spontaneously, especially in roan ponies and cobs. This form of the condition is hereditary. The depigmented areas are usually located around the eyes, muzzle and lips (*Figures 15.24 and*

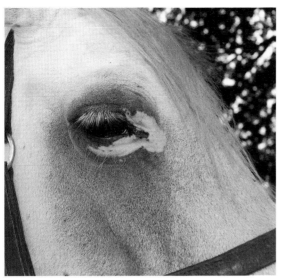

Figure 15.24   *Depigmented area of skin around the eye of a horse with vitiligo*

15.25). Occasionally the vulva, anus, sheath or penis are affected.

Treatment

There is no treatment.

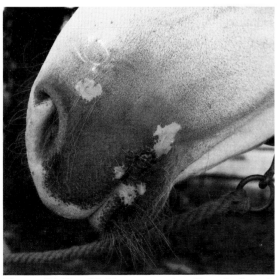

Figure 15.25   *Vitiligo commonly affects the horse's lips and muzzle*

Nodular Skin Disease

Nodular skin disease (*Figure 15.26*) is characterised by raised nodules on the withers, neck, back, chest wall or abdomen.

Causes

The cause is unknown, but as the lesions develop in spring and summer, they may be a reaction to insect bites.

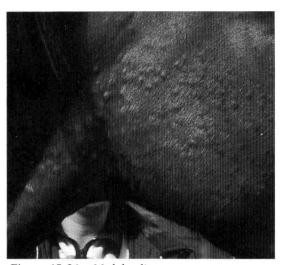

Figure 15.26   *Nodular disease*

Clinical signs

The round, raised nodules are:
- 0.5–5 cm in diameter
- firm to touch
- painless
- non-irritant
- variable in number, from one or two to several hundreds.

There is usually no hair loss, and the nodules may persist for months or years.

Diagnosis

Diagnosis is confirmed by examination of a skin biopsy.

The mass consists of degenerating collagen fibres and numerous eosinophils. Calcium deposits may be found in large or long-standing lesions.

Treatment

The nodules sometimes regress without treatment. In other cases, corticosteroids may be effective.

Surgical excision is necessary for non-responsive or calcified lesions.

Prognosis

The condition does not always respond to medical treatment, and surgical excision is only practical when there are a small number of nodules. The prognosis is therefore guarded.

16 Eye Injury and Disease

Diagnosis and Treatment

The eyes of a horse are relatively prominent and therefore susceptible to injury. If any abnormality is seen, consult your vet at once because early diagnosis and treatment assist healing and minimise the risk of complications. A few examples of eye conditions requiring immediate treatment include:

Torn eyelids

These require prompt and careful suturing. If left to heal on their own, the eyelid margins may become distorted and cause chronic corneal disease.

Corneal abrasions

If corneal abrasions are overlooked or neglected they can develop into deep ulcers. They take a long time to heal and cause permanent scarring.

Inflammation

Where this occurs within the eye immediate treatment is required to relieve the pain and

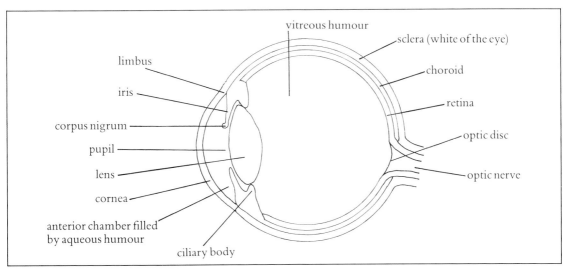

Figure 16.1 *Vertical section through a horse's eye*

keep the damage to a minimum. In cases of recurrent uveitis, prompt treatment slows down the onset of blindness.

Tumours

These are easier to treat and carry a more favourable prognosis when diagnosed early.

Examination of an injured eye

Where a horse is in obvious discomfort with its eyelids tightly closed, *do not* force them open. By trying to do so you could inadvertently apply sufficient pressure to rupture a severely damaged eye.

Leave the examination to the vet who can use topical anaesthesia, nerve blocks and sedatives to relax the horse and alleviate the discomfort. Once the pain is removed, the horse will open its eye and be more amenable to examination.

In addition to looking for external injuries, the vet will also check the internal structures of the eye (*Figure 16.1*) with an ophthalmo-scope. This part of the examination is carried out in a darkened box.

A fluorescent dye may be used to detect ulcers and scratches on the cornea.

How to apply eye ointment

The treatment of many eye injuries and diseases involves frequent application of drops or ointment.

This is not easy if the eye is sore and the horse is uncooperative. Inexpert or careless technique can frighten the horse and cause further damage.

The following tips may help.
1) In cold weather, warm the ointment to body temperature as this makes it easier to apply.
2) Whenever possible, have an assistant to hold the horse.
3) Gently wipe any discharge away using moist cotton wool.
4) Remove the top and hold the tube in your right hand. Position the hand so it rests against the horse's cheek (*Figure 16.2*).
5) With the fingers and thumb of the left hand, gently evert (turn out) the lower

Figure 16.2   *Rest your hand against the horse's cheek when applying eye ointment*

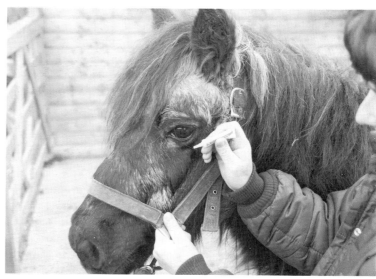

eyelid (*Figure 16.3*). Do not apply unnecessary pressure to the eyeball.

6) Squeeze a line of ointment along the length of the exposed conjunctival sac.

With your right hand fixed firmly against the horse's cheek, there is little danger of the nozzle poking the eye. Your hand will follow any sudden movements of the head.

The use of an indwelling nasolacrimal cannula

Where the horse resents handling of the eye, treatment can be administered through an indwelling nasolacrimal cannula (*Figure 16.4*).

The nasolacrimal duct runs from the inner corner of the eye to an opening on the floor of the nostril. Its function is to drain excess tear film from the eyes.

With the horse sedated, the end of the cannula is passed through a small incision in the skin of the false nostril. It is gently pushed into the opening of the duct and sutured in position.

The remaining length of the cannula is sutured at intervals along the face and neck or taped to the headcollar (*Figures 16.4 and 16.5*).

A head and neck cover made from stretch material can be used to prevent the cannula from catching on projections and being pulled out. Medication can then be administered through the cannula without any handling of the eye.

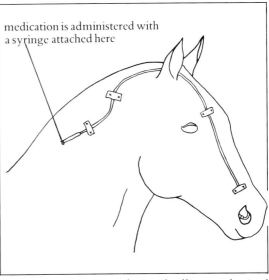

medication is administered with a syringe attached here

Figure 16.4   *Horse with an indwelling nasolacrimal cannula*

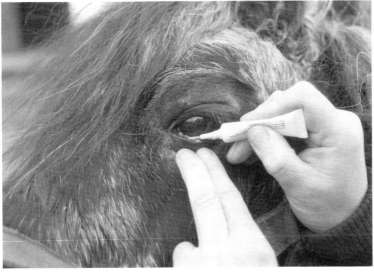

Figure 16.3   *Evert the lower eyelid and squeeze the ointment into the conjunctival sac*

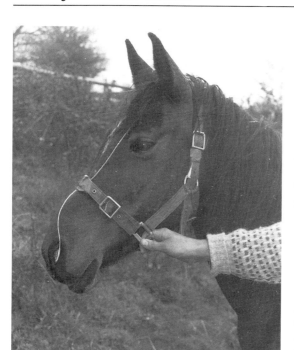

Figure 16.5　*A nasolacrimal cannula sutured to the nostril and taped to the headcollar*

Treatment is continued until the lesion has healed. This can take a few days or several weeks.

Hygiene guidelines

- Always wash your hands before applying treatment.
- Ensure the nozzle of the tube or syringe is not contaminated with dirt or discharge.
- Use a separate tube for each horse to avoid cross-infection.
- Throw away any partly used tubes when the condition has resolved. Treatments must be used within a month of the tube being opened.

Stable management

Exposure to light increases the discomfort experienced by animals with certain eye conditions. Horses with uveitis or corneal erosions, for example, must be kept in a darkened stable. They may be turned out for a couple of hours at night.

Irritation from flies and dust must be kept to a minimum. Hay should be soaked and fed from the floor.

Injuries to the Cornea

The *cornea* is the transparent tissue at the front of the eye. It is very susceptible to injury from twigs and barbed wire.

Corneal injuries are prone to secondary infection by bacteria and fungi which can cause the development of deep, non-healing ulcers.

Inflammation of the cornea is known as *keratitis*. It can be caused by injury, chemical irritants or viral infection.

Clinical signs

The clinical signs will include some of the following.
- Pain. The horse often squints or keeps its eyelids tightly closed (*Figure 16.6*).
- Profuse tear production. If secondary bacterial infection develops, the discharge becomes purulent.
- Irregularities on the normally smooth corneal surface.
- Cloudy, grey-white patches on the cornea.
- Blood vessels growing in from the corneal margin.

Diagnosis

Diagnosis is made following a thorough examination of the eye. This is a good example of a situation where firmly closed eyelids should not be forced open because of the danger of rupturing the eyeball.

Some corneal injuries are readily observed, but very tiny ulcers or abrasions show up more clearly following the application of fluorescein eye drops.

The appearance of the lesion can be suggestive of the cause. For example, superficial keratitis caused by viral infection is characterised by lace-like patterns or a number of tiny ulcers on the cornea.

Swabs or scrapings may be taken from non-healing ulcers and cultured for bacteria or fungi. Antibiotic sensitivity tests can then be performed.

Treatment

Medication in the form of ointments or drops is applied topically several times a day. The type of medication (bactericidal, fungicidal or viricidal) depends on the nature of the lesion. Ointments containing a corticosteroid must not be used unless under direct veterinary supervision as they can delay healing and lead to secondary fungal infection.

Where the horse resists treatment or the lesion is slow to heal, an indwelling nasolacrimal cannula is used.

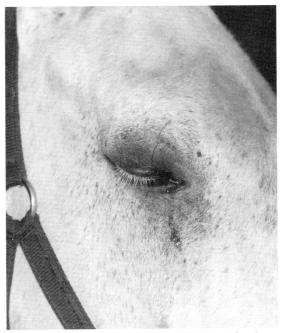

Figure 16.6   *Horses with a corneal injury often keep their eyelids tightly closed*

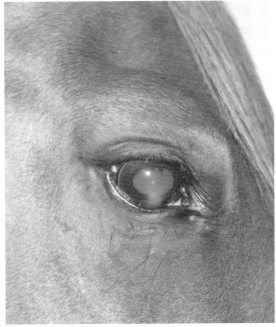

Figure 16.7   *Cloudy area on the cornea. This injury has happened because the horse has a dense cataract and no sight in its eye following several episodes of recurrent uveitis*

Antibiotic or antifungal drugs may also be injected underneath the conjunctiva. They are released slowly onto the eye over a period of several days.

The horse must be kept in a dimly lit box and fed soaked hay from the floor to prevent further irritation.

Prognosis

Superficial injuries that are correctly managed heal within a few days.

Deep ulcers take much longer to heal and usually leave a scar.

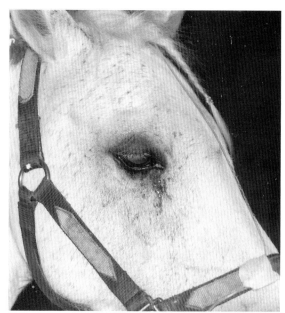

Figure 16.8   *Conjunctivitis*

Conjunctivitis

Conjunctivitis (*Figure 16.8*) is inflammation of the conjunctiva.

The conjunctiva is the moist, pink mucous membrane that lines the eyelids and attaches them to the eyeball. It also covers the third eyelid which is located at the inner corner of the eye.

Causes

The causes of conjunctivitis include:
- wind
- dust
- fly irritation
- allergy (e.g. pollen)
- trauma
- foreign bodies
- eyelid deformities
- bacterial infection.

Conjunctivitis may also be a symptom of respiratory virus infection.

Clinical signs

The condition tends to affect both eyes unless it is caused by trauma or a foreign body.

The symptoms include:
- pain
- excessive tear production
- a tendency to keep the eyelids half closed
- redness and/or swelling of the conjunctiva (*Figure 16.9*)
- a discharge of pus if secondary bacterial infection occurs
- the development of follicles of lymphoid tissue.

Diagnosis

Diagnosis is made on the clinical signs. The conjunctival sac must be examined thoroughly to rule out the presence of a foreign body.

Anaesthetic drops instilled into the eye numb the conjunctiva and make the examination easier.

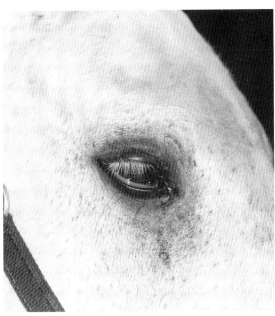

Figure 16.9   *Conjunctivitis: note the conjunctival swelling*

A fluorescent dye may be used to check for corneal damage. Any abrasions are stained a brilliant green.

Treatment

Antibiotic and corticosteroid ointment is applied three times a day to control the infection and inflammation.

Where there is a corneal injury in addition to conjunctival inflammation, *remember* that treatments containing a corticosteroid should not be used. These cases are treated with antibiotic ointment or drops.

Cataract

A cataract is an opacity of the lens. Many are small and non-progressive, causing little, if any, impairment of vision.

Other cataracts are progressive. They affect the horse's sight and can eventually lead to blindness.

Causes

Cataracts may be congenital (i.e. present at birth) or acquired as a result of injury, disease or old age.

Clinical signs

Horses with small, non-progressive cataracts show no clinical signs. Many cataracts are only discovered when a horse is vetted for a prospective purchaser.

Where cataracts are causing a progressive loss of sight, the signs include:

- stumbling
- walking into objects
- an abnormal number of facial injuries
- sudden shying.

Diagnosis

Diagnosis is made by examination of the eye with an ophthalmoscope.

Treatment

There is no treatment.

Prognosis

It is impossible to predict the speed at which a cataract will develop from a single examination. The clinical findings must be recorded and the horse should be re-examined at 3–6 monthly intervals.

Affected mares can be used for breeding as the chance of cataracts being inherited is remote.

The Partially-sighted horse

Sight may be lost because of a cataract, a serious injury (*Figure 16.10*) or if an eye has to be removed (*Figure 16.11*), e.g. to prevent the spread of a tumour. These horses will require careful management.

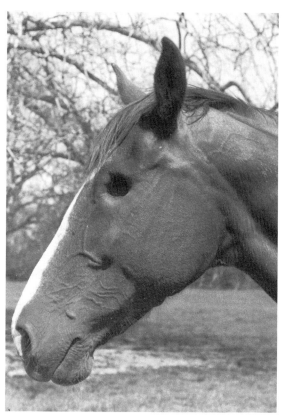

Figure 16.11   *A one-eyed mare, now retired to stud*

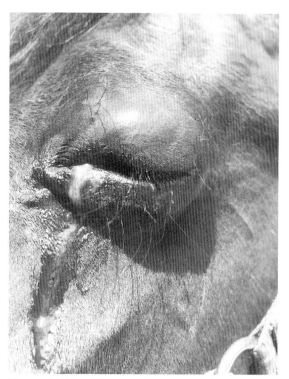

Figure 16.10   *This mare has a ruptured eye, requiring immediate surgical removal*

Management

The partially-sighted horse should be approached and handled with particular care so that it is not startled.

When its sight is lost suddenly, the horse may find it more difficult to adjust than when the loss of sight is gradual.

Provided that they are of a sensible disposition, one-eyed horses are capable of most activities.

N.B. When there is loss of vision or complete blindness in one eye, the other eye must be regularly checked for any sign of disease.

Recurrent Uveitis

Recurrent uveitis is a serious disease that can affect one or both eyes.

The iris, ciliary body and the choroid (collectively known as the uveal tract), become inflamed. With each episode there is further damage and the changes within the eye may lead to blindness.

The disease is also known as periodic ophthalmia or moon blindness. Fortunately it is not common.

Causes

The cause of the condition has not been conclusively identified. It may be an allergic reaction to an infection with leptospirosis or the worm *Onchocerca cervicalis*.

Clinical signs

The symptoms develop very quickly over a period of a few hours. They include:
- pain
- closed eyelids and obvious discomfort in bright light
- increased tear production
- cloudiness of the cornea
- constriction of the pupil
- a collection of white blood cells and other debris in the anterior chamber (between the cornea and the iris)
- a dull appearance of the iris which never regains its normal lustre.

The inflammation usually lasts for 7–10 days. The interval between the attacks may be days, weeks, months or years.

Over a period of time the eyeball becomes smaller. Retinal degeneration and cataract formation cause progressive loss of sight.

Treatment

The aim of treatment is to reduce the pain and inflammation. It should be started as soon as the symptoms develop to minimise the damage within the eye.
- Atropine drops are used to dilate (open) the pupil. This is necessary because the inflamed iris can become stuck to the front of the lens while the pupil is constricted.

   In some cases the pupil does not fully dilate. It acquires an irregular outline because parts of the iris remain attached to the lens.

   When adhesions between the iris and the lens are broken down, pigmented deposits are often left on the lens capsule
- Corticosteroid drops are applied to relieve the inflammation.
- Systemic non-steroidal anti-inflammatory drugs, e.g. phenylbutazone or flunixin meglumine, are also used.
- The horse must be kept in a darkened box for the following reasons:
  – light increases the pain especially when the pupil has been dilated by atropine
  – darkness encourages the pupil to dilate naturally.

Prognosis

The prognosis is extremely guarded. It is not possible to predict the frequency of attacks or how quickly the horse will lose its sight.

Eye Tumours

Sarcoids and squamous cell carcinomas are the tumours that most commonly affect the eye.

Sarcoid

Sarcoids often occur on the upper eyelid. They grow fairly rapidly and tend to ulcerate (*Figure 16.12*).

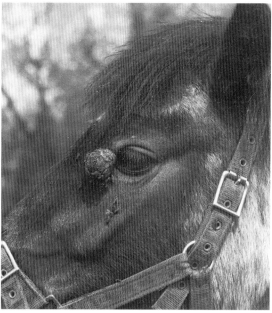

Figure 16.12 *Ulcerated sarcoid attached to the upper eyelid of a pony*

For treatment of sarcoids to be successful, all the tumour tissue must be removed or destroyed. This is simplest, and has the least risk of complications, when the tumour is small.

Squamous Cell Carcinoma

Squamous cell carcinomas occur on:
- the conjunctiva lining the eyelids
- the third eyelid
- the limbus (the junction between the transparent cornea and the white sclera of the eye).

The tumour tissue is pink, moist and granular in appearance. Affected eyes may have a thick, mucopurulent discharge.

Early recognition and treatment is essential as the tumour can spread to local lymph nodes and salivary glands.

Treatment involves surgical removal, followed by cryosurgery or radiation therapy.

17 The Reproductive System

Castration

Castration or gelding involves removal of the horse's testicles.

This operation is carried out to make the horse:
- sterile
- more placid, especially in the presence of mares.

Preparing for the operation

A number of factors should be considered when making the arrangements for a horse to be gelded.

These include:

Timing

Horses can be gelded at any age. The most popular time is between 1–2 years.

The operation should take place in the spring, autumn or winter when there are relatively few flies.

Location

The horse may be gelded in a field with a good grass cover.

Alternatively, a stable with a *clean* bed of dust free straw or paper may be used. Wood shavings are not suitable as tiny chips can enter the wound and cause problems later. The bed should be prepared well in advance so the atmosphere is not dusty when the operation takes place.

The horse

The horse should be:
- in good health; if he is off colour or in poor condition, the operation should be postponed
- clean and dry
- starved if the operation is being done under general anaesthesia
- calm and relaxed
- well handled.

Veterinary requirements

The vet will need:
- a competent handler to hold the horse
- a clean bucket of warm water.

Procedure

The vet will commence with a preoperative examination of the horse, to ensure it is in good health.

The scrotal region is carefully palpated to check that both testicles are present.

The vet will also check for any signs of an inguinal hernia. This occurs when the inguinal ring which separates the abdominal cavity and the scrotum is larger than normal. Loops of bowel may periodically enter the scrotal sac. If a hernia goes undetected, the bowel can become strangulated or prolapse through the castration wound.

Anaesthesia

Horses can be gelded under local or general anaesthesia. The vet will discuss this with the horse's owner in advance.

With local anaesthesia, the horse is sedated but remains standing. A twitch is usually applied.

Where only one testicle has descended or other problems are suspected, the procedure is carried out under general anaesthesia.

The operation

1) The vet will wash the area with an antiseptic solution.
2) The scrotum is incised. Emasculators are used to remove the testicles and crush the cord.
3) Tetanus antitoxin and antibiotics are given.
4) Non-steroidal anti-inflammatory drugs, e.g. phenylbutazone, may be used to minimise the swelling and discomfort.

Aftercare

The horse should be turned out into a clean, grassy field as soon as it is fully conscious and the bleeding has stopped. This helps to keep the swelling to a minimum.

The horse should then be checked for complications at regular intervals throughout the day and over the next week.

Possible complications

Haemorrhage

In most cases, blood will drip from the wound for a few minutes. This is to be expected and is no cause for concern.

However, if the dripping persists or blood runs from the wound in a continuous stream, contact your vet.

Swelling/infection

All horses experience some swelling following castration. It is usually controlled by turning the horse out and giving in-hand or lungeing exercise.

If the swelling seems excessive or does not begin to reduce after four days, call the vet. It may be due to infection and the horse will require a course of antibiotics.

Prolapse of loops of gut

When loops of gut hang from the castration wound, this is an emergency.

Request immediate veterinary help and try to keep the gut off the floor using a clean sheet or towel.

If the gut is not too badly damaged, the horse may be saved by immediate surgery.

Scrotal abscess

A painful swelling develops within two months of the surgery. It may burst spontaneously or require lancing.

Champignon

A mushroom-shaped growth of proud flesh protrudes from the scrotal wound. This develops within a few weeks of the operation. It must be surgically removed.

Scirrhous cord

This condition occurs years after the horse has been gelded. A swelling develops in the groin region and there may be several skin openings discharging pus.

Treatment involves surgical excision of the infected tissue and a long course of antibiotics. If the infection has spread into the abdomen, the prognosis is hopeless.

Cystic ends

A fluid-filled cyst may develop in the scrotum some months or years after castration. The swelling can make the horse look as though it is still entire. The cyst is painless and no treatment is necessary.

simple blood test can be used to determine whether a testis is present.

Castration

When a horse is found to have a single testicle at the preoperative examination, there are two possible courses of action.
- In young animals the operation may be postponed in the hope that an inguinal testicle will descend over the next few months.
- Arrangements can be made to perform the operation under general anaesthesia. The horse should be taken to a veterinary hospital as the surgery may involve exploration of the abdomen.

A single scrotal testis is never removed on its own.

Breeding

Cryptorchid animals should not be used for breeding as the condition is hereditary.

The Cryptorchid Horse (Rig)

Cryptorchid is the name given to an animal with one or both testes retained in the inguinal region or the abdomen. Cryptorchid horses are known as 'rigs'.

Retained testes produce hormones and cause the horse to behave like a stallion. If the history of a particular animal is unknown and its behaviour gives cause for concern, a

Introduction to Breeding

There are three questions for those owners considering breeding from a mare.
- *Is she suitable for breeding?*
  Traits such as conformation and temperament are highly heritable and should be important considerations when selecting the mare and stallion. Mares should be selected for quality of type or performance and not simply because they are unsuitable

for any other purpose. Mares with serious conformational defects should not be bred from.
- *Are suitable facilities available?*
Consideration must also be given to the facilities required. You will need a foaling box and suitably fenced, good quality pasture. Ideally, the field should be shared with other mares and foals.
- *Can I afford it?*
Stud fees, livery charges and veterinary bills can add up to a substantial sum and there is no guarantee that a healthy foal will be produced.

General information

Most mares have a 21 day oestrous cycle. This is divided into:
- oestrus (4–6 days)
- dioestrus (15–17) days.

Oestrus

The mare is receptive to the stallion and is said to be 'in season'. Typical signs of oestrus include:
- adopting the urinating stance and passing small amounts of bright yellow urine
- everting the vulval lips to expose the clitoris (winking).

During this time a follicle on the ovary increases in size and ruptures to release an egg (ovulation). The mare normally ovulates 24–48 hours before the end of oestrus.
The maturation of the follicle can be monitored by the vet on successive rectal examinations.

Dioestrus

The mare behaves aggressively towards the stallion. She puts her ears back, swishes her tail and may squeal or lash out.

Control of the oestrous cycle

The mare has a seasonal breeding period which is influenced by factors such as daylight length and temperature.

Between the months of October/November and February/March most mares stop having oestrous cycles and their ovaries become small and inactive.

The mare is most fertile in April, May, June and July. However, there is considerable individual variation between mares. During spring and early autumn, some will ovulate without showing oestrous behaviour. Others will have long periods of oestrous behaviour in the spring, but fail to ovulate.

The oestrous cycles are under hormonal control. When problems arise, oestrus or ovulation can sometimes be induced by hormone treatments.

Gestation length

The gestation (pregnancy) length is 11 months (340 days), but it is not unusual for a mare to foal up to three weeks late. One per cent of pregnancies last for 12 months.

Stallion selection

The choice of stallion should be made after considering the following factors.
- Conformation – which must compensate for any minor conformational weaknesses of the mare.
- Soundness and freedom from hereditary conditions.
- Performance record – achievements during his working career.
- Temperament – ideally calm and kind.

- Size.
- Fertility record – a mare with a history of infertility should be sent to a highly fertile stallion.
- Cost and terms of stud fee.
- Distance away.

It is worth travelling to view one or two selected stallions rather than opting for the convenience of the closest one. Try to see some of the stallion's offspring.

Artificial Insemination (AI)

AI is becoming increasingly available for non-Thoroughbred breeds.

Semen is collected in an artificial vagina and inseminated into the mare by the vet.

Semen may be used fresh, chilled or frozen. For it to be suitable for AI, it must be:
- from a high class stallion
- of excellent quality
- able to withstand the chilling or freezing process.

Survival time

Chilled semen will keep for up to 12 hours when transported in special containers. Frozen semen keeps indefinitely, but is only suitable for young, fertile mares.

Advantages

The advantages of AI are:
- it prevents the spread of venereal (sexually transmitted) disease

- fewer bacteria enter the uterus than with natural service
- there is no risk of kick injuries to the stallion and the mare
- in expert hands it increases the chance of pregnancy; the mare is regularly examined and semen is inseminated just before ovulation
- mares and foals do not need to travel long distances to the stud.

Disadvantages

AI is expensive. The mare requires frequent examinations by an experienced stud vet. If the mare does not ovulate when expected, the insemination must be repeated at intervals until she does.

Veterinary Care of the Brood Mare

The vet is usually consulted at several stages of the breeding programme, e.g.:
- gynaecological examination prior to covering
- pregnancy diagnosis
- vaccination
- post-foaling checks.

Gynaecological examination

The purpose of the gynaecological examination is to check for any problems that could affect the mare's ability to conceive. It includes:
- inspection of the vulva, vagina and cervix
- rectal palpation of the uterus and ovaries.

The examination will reveal any major differences from the normal (*Figures 17.1 and 17.2*). It also gives an indication of whether the mare is cycling and the stage of the cycle.

Preparation

Where purpose-built stocks are not available, the mare should be examined in a stable. She must wear a bridle and a clean tail bandage.

The vet will require:

- a bucket of warm water
- two assistants – one to hold the mare and another to lift the tail out of the way and pass the swabs
- power for the scanner.

It may be necessary to apply a twitch for the examination.

Assessment

Poor vulval conformation allows air to enter the vagina and uterus. This can lead to infertility and is treated by a *Caslick's operation*, i.e.

suturing the upper part of the vulval lips together under local anaesthesia.

The vulva must be opened before the mare foals. It can be done by the vet a few days prior to foaling, or by the stud personnel as the mare enters second-stage labour.

Swabs and smears

Swabs and smears are taken to ensure that the mare is not suffering from a bacterial infection of the genital tract. An infected mare will not conceive, so covering her is a waste of time and money. More importantly, a mare with venereal disease will infect the stallion and any mares he subsequently covers.

Maiden mares are not exempt from uterine infection and should also be swabbed.

There are two types of swab.

Clitoral swab

A clitoral swab may be taken at any stage of the oestrous cycle.

A narrow-tipped swab is introduced into

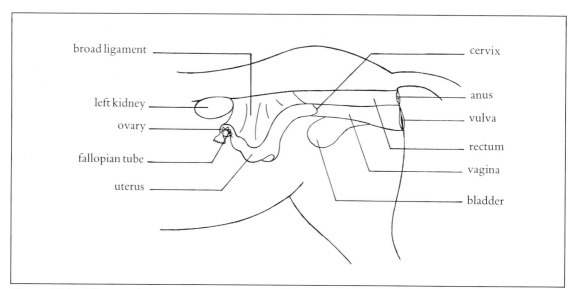

Figure 17.1   *The reproductive tract of the mare*

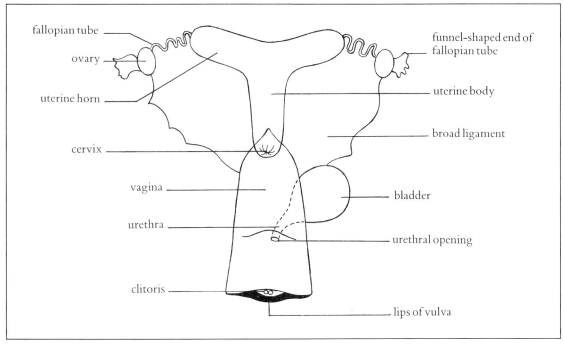

Figure 17.2 *The reproductive tract of the mare – with the vulva and vagina opened*

the clitoral sinuses and rolled around the clitoral fossa. It is then cultured for bacteria that cause venereal disease. These include *Tayorella equigenitalis*, the organism responsible for Contagious Equine Metritis (CEM), *Klebsiella pneumoniae* and *Pseudomonas aeruginosa*. The CEM culture takes six days.

Many studs require a copy of the culture results before accepting the mare onto the premises.

Endometrial swab and smear

Endometrial swabs and smears are taken from the inner lining of the uterus (endometrium). They can only be taken when the mare is in season and the cervix is relaxed.

Endometrial swab

A sterile swab is passed via a speculum,

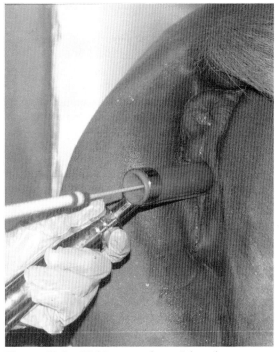

Figure 17.3 *Taking an endometrial swab*

through the cervix into the uterus (*Figure 17.3*).

The swab is then cultured for 48 hours. If bacteria that are known to cause uterine infection are grown, a sensitivity test is carried out. The mare is then treated with the appropriate antibiotics.

Endometrial smear

A sterile swab is passed through the cervix and gently rubbed against the endometrium. The swab is then rolled onto a slide coated with gelatin. Cells from the endometrium are transferred to the slide which is stained and examined under a microscope.

If neutrophils are seen amongst the endometrial cells, this indicates acute inflammation of the endometrium (endometritis). It is usually the result of infection.

Treatment of endometritis

Where the laboratory results show the mare is suffering from endometritis, she will be treated with intrauterine antibiotics for a period of 3–5 days.

In some cases a special intrauterine infuser is used. The antibiotic can then be administered by stud personnel or the owner. This device will only stay in place when the mare is no longer in season and the cervix has tightened up.

A second swab and smear must be taken early in the following oestrus. If the treatment has been successful and there is no evidence of endometritis, the mare can be covered.

Treatment of venereal disease

Treatment of diseases such as CEM requires:
- intrauterine infusions of antibiotic
- thorough cleaning and topical antibiotic treatment of the clitoris.

Treatment can be expensive as some infections are difficult to clear up. Surgical removal of the clitoris may be necessary with stubborn cases.

Endometrial biopsy

If the mare fails to conceive, or the swabs and smears reveal persistent or recurrent infection, an endometrial biopsy may be taken. This is done during dioestrus.

Biopsy forceps are passed through the cervix and a small piece of endometrium is removed and sent to a laboratory. Examination of the tissue under the microscope reveals the extent of any inflammatory or degenerative changes in the endometrium. Treatment can then be recommended and a prognosis for successful breeding is given.

A second biopsy is taken one month later to assess the results of the treatment.

18 Pregnancy

Pregnancy Diagnosis

A number of procedures are used to confirm that a mare is in foal (*Figure 18.1*)

Rectal palpation

This can be done at any stage of pregnancy from 17 days onwards. The vet assesses the tone, size and position of the uterus which change as the pregnancy advances. The foal may be felt from around day 200.

When a mare is examined in the early stages of pregnancy, the cervix is inspected through a speculum. It is usually much whiter and more tightly closed than the cervix of a non–pregnant mare.

However, the rectal findings during early pregnancy are frequently inconclusive. A definite diagnosis can be obtained from an ultrasound scan or a re-examination at a later date.

Ultrasound scanning

An ultrasound scanner is used for pregnancy diagnosis and the assessment of early fetal growth from 17 days onwards. It is the most reliable method of detecting unwanted twin pregnancies.

Method

The rectum is emptied of faeces. A probe is introduced and advanced until it lies over the uterus. It is moved from side to side, passing

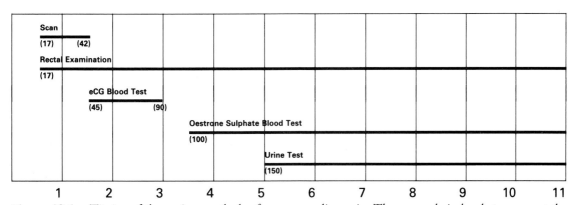

Figure 18.1   *Timing of the various methods of pregnancy diagnosis. The numerals in brackets represent the number of days after conception. The numerals below the baseline represent the time in months*

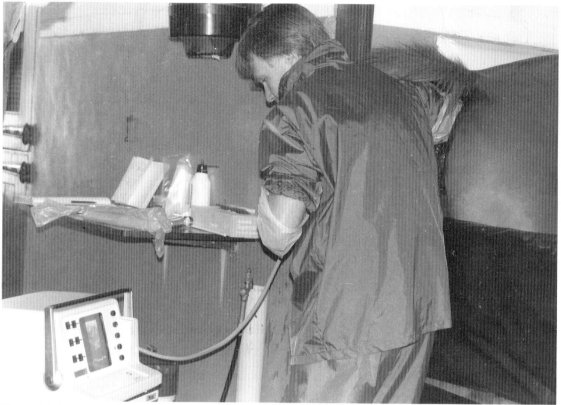

Figure 18.2   *A mare being scanned*

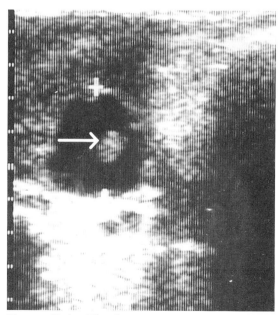

Figure 18.3   *The fetus is seen as a white speck (marked by the arrow) within a black circle on the scanner*

over the uterine horns and the ovaries (*Figure 18.2*).

An image is produced on a screen. If the mare is pregnant, the fetus is seen as a small, white speck within a circular black area (*Figure 18.3*).

When a mare is scanned early in pregnancy, the procedure is repeated at 42 days. This is to check:

- fetal growth
- for early fetal death
- that a second fetus – too small to be seen on the first examination – has not developed.

Blood tests

Equine chorionic gonadotrophin (eCG)

From days 45–90, a blood sample may be taken and tested for the presence of eCG.

This is produced by structures called endometrial cups which form when fetal cells invade the endometrium.

The test is 90 per cent accurate. A few mares produce false negatives, but inaccuracies more commonly involve false positives. This is because eCG continues to be produced if the fetus dies.

Oestrone sulphate

Oestrone sulphate is produced by the fetus and can be detected in the serum of pregnant mares from day 100.

Urine tests

Oestrogens produced by the placenta and the fetus are present in urine from 150 days to full term.

Management of the In-Foal Mare

Long, tiring journeys should be avoided between 20–45 days after conception. When a mare has been transported a considerable distance to stud, it is advisable to leave her there until pregnancy has been confirmed at 42 days.

Care during pregnancy

Once the pregnant mare is home she will require:
- daily inspection
- regular hoof care
- correct feeding
- regular worming

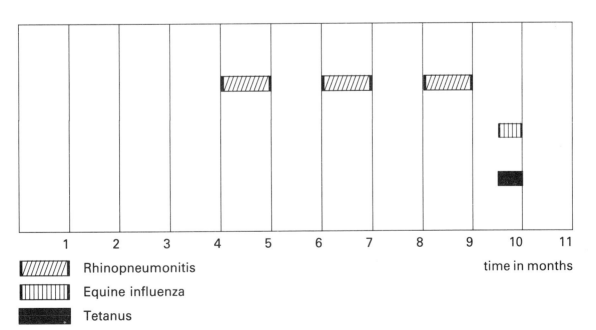

Figure 18.4   *Timing of vaccinations for brood mares*

- teeth rasping
- vaccination (*Figure 18.4*)
  - *influenza and tetanus*: a booster 3–6 weeks before foaling gives the foal maximum protection
  - *equine rhinopneumonitis (virus abortion)*: this vaccination is recommended during months five, seven and nine of pregnancy.

Exercise

This depends on many factors such as size, age, condition and fitness of the mare and the weight of the rider.

Strenuous exercise should be discontinued from the sixth month of gestation.

The brood mare should be turned out each day.

Abortion

Even with the best of care, 10 per cent of mares do not carry their foals to term. Abortion is defined as the loss of the foal and its membranes before the 300th day of gestation.

Causes

- Infection:
  - bacterial
  - fungal
  - viral (EHV–1).
- Twins: the placenta is rarely able to nourish two foals to full term.
- Maternal stress, e.g.:
  - malnutrition
  - pain
  - a high temperature

  - emotional disturbance from weaning or management changes
  - travelling.
- Developmental abnormalities in the foal, placenta or umbilical cord.
- Twisting of the umbilical cord.
- Uterine abnormality.

Because EHV–1 is so infectious and can cause multiple abortions within a group of mares, tests should be carried out to eliminate it from the list of possible causes.

If a mare aborts:
- contact the vet immediately
- isolate the mare in a stable
- put the fetus and membranes in a leak-proof container
- disinfect any areas likely to be contaminated by fetal fluids.

Follow the Code of Practice drawn up by the Thoroughbred Breeders' Association. (See Equine Herpes Virus 1, Chapter 14.)

Preparation for Foaling

The mare should be moved to the foaling premises six weeks before she is due to foal. This gives her time to settle in and to acquire an immunity to disease-producing organisms in the new environment. She will produce protective antibodies which are passed on to the foal in the colostrum.

For an average-size mare, the foaling box should measure 4.5 m × 4.5 m. A clean, deep bed of good quality straw should be provided. Shavings are not suitable as they can block the nostrils of a newborn foal.

A power point and a means of providing a sick foal with warmth should be available.

The last four weeks

Mammary development

The udder of the mare begins to enlarge approximately four weeks before foaling. Most of the development takes place in the last two weeks when both the udder and ventral abdomen can become oedematous.

Drops of dried colostrum may accumulate as waxy deposits on the teats 1–4 days before foaling.

These signs should not be regarded as a reliable indication that foaling is imminent. Some mares show very little change until the last few hours while others run milk for days or weeks before foaling.

Milk strip tests

Over the last three weeks, the composition of the mammary secretion changes. A special kit is available for use near term to predict whether the mare is likely to foal in the next 24 hours.

Vulval relaxation

Shortly before birth, the vulva lengthens and appears slightly swollen.

Foaling

As the foaling date approaches, the mare should be kept under supervision at all times. She should be checked regularly at night.

The observer should be familiar with the course of a normal foaling and call the vet if a problem occurs.

Sitting up can cause the loss of much sleep, especially if the mare foals three weeks late.

Foaling alarms can be attached to a surcingle and breast plate. When the mare begins to sweat, a bleeper is triggered.

First-stage labour

During first-stage labour the mare experiences discomfort from uterine contractions. The signs include:
- restlessness
- sweating
- pawing the ground
- looking round at the flanks
- milk spurting from the teats.

The periods of discomfort are separated by periods of calm. Maiden mares may roll or become quite upset. The length of first-stage labour is extremely variable.

Second-stage labour

Second-stage labour lasts for an average of 20 minutes.

It begins when the placenta ruptures and a large quantity of yellowish-brown fluid is released.

Most mares then lie on their sides and begin to strain. If the mare has a sutured vulva which has not already been opened, it must be cut at this stage.

After 5–10 minutes, a white membrane called the amnion appears between the vulval lips. In a normal foaling the front feet are delivered first, followed closely by the muzzle.

The mare continues to strain vigorously until the foal's hips have been delivered. She will then stop straining but stay lying down for up to 20 minutes.

Do not disturb her, especially for the first few minutes after foaling as blood is still passing from the placenta to the foal. It is quite normal for the foal's hind limbs to remain inside the vagina and unless the amnion is blocking the foal's nostrils, no interference is necessary.

The umbilical cord breaks when the mare stands or the foal struggles to get up. The foal's navel should then be dressed with iodine or antibiotic powder/spray.

Third-stage labour

The placenta is normally expelled within an hour of the foal being born. The mare may go down and experience colicky pain as it is delivered.

If the placenta has not been expelled within six hours, call the vet.

Complications associated with retained placenta include:
- acute metritis (infection of the uterus)
- toxaemia
- laminitis.

Post-Foaling Checks

These checks are very important.

The afterbirth

Spread the placenta out and make sure it is complete. If in doubt, consult someone with more experience or the vet.

The foal

Most foals are on their feet within an hour of birth.

The foal should search for the teats and suck vigorously within two hours of birth. It then feeds at 30–60 minute intervals.

Veterinary attention should be sought if:
- the foal is not standing within two hours
- it shows little, or no, inclination to suck in the first three hours.

The importance of colostrum

Colostrum is the thick yellow milk that is in the udder when the foal is born. It contains antibodies that give protection against infection and must be sucked by the foal in the first few hours of life.

If the mare runs milk prior to foaling, this valuable protection is lost. Contact the vet or the stud to see if colostrum can be obtained from elsewhere.

Veterinary inspection

A veterinary inspection of the newborn foal is recommended. Any problems or weaknesses can then be detected and dealt with before complications arise.

The vet may give the foal tetanus antitoxin and antibiotic injections and take a blood sample to measure IgG levels. This test is used to check the foal has received sufficient immunity from the colostrum.

19 Veterinary Procedures

Vetting a Horse

It is advisable to have any horse examined by a veterinary surgeon prior to purchase. With their experience and specialist instruments, vets are often able to detect problems that are not immediately obvious to the owner or the prospective purchaser.

A veterinary certificate *Figure 19.1* may be necessary to obtain insurance cover. The procedure is laid down in a Joint Memorandum prepared by the Royal College of Veterinary Surgeons and the British Veterinary Association entitled *The Examination of Horses on Behalf of a Purchaser*. It is very thorough, taking one and a half to two hours.

The examination is divided into five stages. On completion of the examination, the vet lists any defects noted and will give an opinion as to the suitability of the horse for its intended use.

Contacting a veterinary practice

If you are not registered with a practice, or are buying a horse too far away for your own vet to examine, you will need to contact a new practice. Either ask friends, or your own vet, to recommend a practice, or contact the vendor's practice and ask them for the names of other equine practices in the area.

Vets are understandably reluctant to carry out purchase examinations on horses belonging to their own clients. If you and the vendor both use the same vet, you may need to find someone else to do the vetting.

Initial briefing

It is very important that the intended use of the animal and the rider's level of experience are known to the vet before the examination takes place. Without this information the vet will be unable to offer an opinion on suitability. Wherever possible, the purchaser should attend the vetting. A great deal can be learned about the temperament of the horse during the examination. Any points raised by the vet can be discussed before the final decision is made.

Preparation for the vetting

Exercise and stabling

The horse or pony should be stabled the night before the examination and not exercised prior to the vet's visit. This increases the likelihood of respiratory allergies or slight stiffness being detected.

Grooming

The horse must be clean and dry but the feet

Figure 19.1
*The vetting
certificate*

CERTIFICATE OF VETERINARY EXAMINATION OF A HORSE ON BEHALF OF A PURCHASER

NAME OF HORSE (OR BREEDING)	BREED OR TYPE	COLOUR	SEX	AGE OR YEAR OF BIRTH
				★ BY DENTITION ★ Delete as
				★ BY DOCUMENTATION appropriate

NOTES ON WARRANTY:

If a Purchaser wishes to obtain a warranty covering such matters as height, freedom from vices, temperament, the non-administration of drugs prior to examination, or the animal's existing performance as a hunter, show-jumper, riding pony, eventer etc., he is advised to seek such warranty in writing from the vendor, as these are matters between vendor and purchaser and are not the responsibility of the veterinary surgeon.

N.B. This certificate does not cover an examination for pregnancy.

INSTRUCTIONS
1. WRITTEN DESCRIPTION SHOULD BE TYPED OR WRITTEN IN BLOCK CAPITALS
2. WRITTEN DESCRIPTION AND DIAGRAM SHOULD AGREE
3. ALL WHITE MARKINGS SHOULD BE HATCHED IN RED
4. WHORLS MUST BE SHOWN THUS 'X' AND DESCRIBED BELOW IN DETAIL

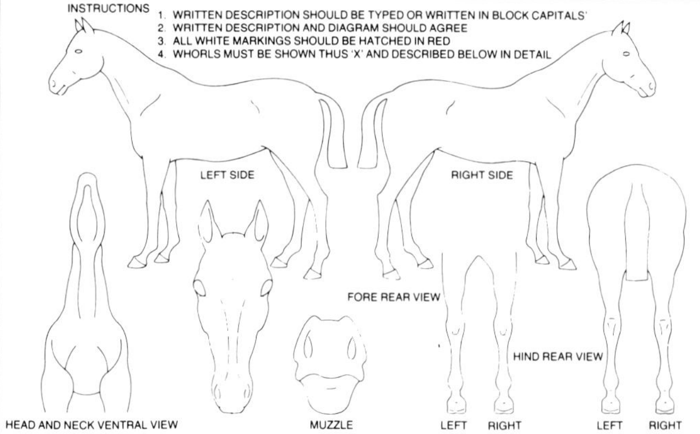

LEFT SIDE   RIGHT SIDE

FORE REAR VIEW

HIND REAR VIEW

HEAD AND NECK VENTRAL VIEW   MUZZLE   LEFT   RIGHT   LEFT   RIGHT

IDENTIFICATION:

Head: ....

Neck: ....

Limbs: L.F. ....
            R.F. ....
            L.H. ....
            R.H. ....
Body: ....

Acquired Marks/Brands: ....

REPORT: This is to certify that at the request of (Name & Address) ....

I have examined the horse described above, the property of (Name & Address) ....

AT (Place of Examination) .... Time and Date of Examination..............................
This clinical examination was carried out substantially in accordance with the standard procedure recommended by the **RCVS** and the **BVA** (Joint Memorandum on the Examination of Horses 1976 revised 1985). The examination is conducted in five stages as set out below.
I cannot find any trace of clinical signs of disease, injury or physical abnormality other than those here recorded:
Signs of disease or injury and other observations: ....

★Radiological or specialised techniques included additional to standard procedure .... Report appended **YES / NO** ★

OPINION: ★(a) On this examination I find no trace of clinical signs of disease, injury or physical abnormality likely to affect the animal's usefulness for ....

★(b) In my opinion on this examination the conditions set out above are not likely to affect the animal's usefulness for ....
★(c) In my opinion on this examination this animal is not suitable for purchase for ....
The opinion herein before expressed is based solely on the clinical examination conducted substantially in accordance with the aforesaid procedure and is made and given subject to the qualification that the said animal may be presently subject to some previously administered drug or medicament intended to or having the effect of masking or concealing some disease, injury or physical abnormality which could otherwise presently be clinically discoverable.
Owing to ....
It was not possible to carry out stage(s) ....of the standard procedure recommended by the **RCVS** and the **BVA** (Joint Memorandum on the Examination of Horses 1976 revised 1985). My opinion is therefore subject to my having been able to carry out a partial examination only and I have been unable to ascertain whether any clinical signs of disease, injury or abnormality would have manifested themselves in the course of that part/those parts of the standard procedure which I was unable to carry out.

THE EXAMINATION: Veterinarians have developed a general routine of examination designed to detect clinical signs of disease and injury. The examination is conducted in five stages

1. Preliminary examination   2. Trotting up   3. Strenuous exercise
4. A period of rest   5. The second trot up and foot examination.
All stages should be completed but if this has not been possible it should be made clear on the certificate in what way the examination has been varied and that any opinions are based on this restricted examination.
Approximate age may be determined by dentition or by documentation.

Veterinarians Name: ....   Address: ....
(IN BLOCK CAPITALS)   ....

Signed: ....   Date of Signature: ....
★DELETE AS APPROPRIATE

should not be oiled. The horse should be well shod or the vetting may have to be postponed.

Rider and assistant

The vendor should provide a competent rider to exercise the horse. An assistant should be available throughout the examination to hold or lead the horse when required.

Facilities

Suitable facilities for exercise must be available. Waterlogged fields, hillsides, and hard rutted surfaces are unsuitable for stage three of the examination.

If necessary, the horse should be transported elsewhere. These arrangements need to be made beforehand to avoid wasting time.

A dark loosebox is required for examination of the eyes.

The vetting procedure

The examination is divided into five stages:
1) Preliminary examination
2) Trotting up
3) Strenuous exercise
4) A period of rest
5) Second trot and foot examination.

The standard vetting procedure does not include:
- x-rays
- endoscopy
- blood tests.

Permission must be obtained from the vendor before these can be carried out.

It also excludes:
- exact height measurement
- pregnancy testing

- a warranty of freedom from vices
- performance records.

If these are important considerations, a written warranty should be sought from the vendor. It is also advisable to obtain details of the horse's vaccination and worming history.

1) Preliminary examination

The horse is observed at rest in the stable. Its condition and resting respiratory movements are noted. The horse is then thoroughly and methodically examined. The tests include the following.
- Listening to the heart and lungs with a stethoscope. It is important to be as quiet as possible during this part of the examination.
- Inspection of the teeth for:
  - an estimation of age
  - alignment
  - abnormal wear
  - the presence of wolf teeth
  - sharp edges
  - any other abnormalities.

  The teeth usually provide a fairly accurate guide to the horse's age up to seven years. After this time, ageing by dentition is less reliable.
- Examination of the eyes with a pen torch and ophthalmoscope to detect any abnormalities.
- Checking the body and limbs. The hands are run over the horse's body and every part is carefully palpated and inspected. Any abnormalities or areas of particular sensitivity are recorded.
- Squeezing the feet with hoof testers to check for any tenderness. Hoof conformation and condition is noted.
- Flexing each limb to ensure there is no pain or restriction of movement.

The horse is now taken outside and inspected in daylight. Conformation is assessed and the approximate height is recorded with the horse standing square on a level surface.

2) *Trotting up and flexion tests*

This part of the examination must be carried out on a hard, level surface. The horse should wear a bridle if examined on the road.
a) The horse is walked in a straight line away from the vet for 20 m, then turned and walked back.
b) The horse is trotted away for 30–40 m and trotted back. The handler should run beside the horse's shoulder and allow unrestricted movement of the head.
c) Each limb in turn is held in a flexed position for a full minute. The horse is asked to move off in trot. Stiffness or lameness is suggestive of joint disease and a variety of other problems.

If the horse passes these checks, stage three is commenced.

3) *Strenuous exercise*

The amount of exercise depends on the age and fitness of the horse, its anticipated use and the facilities available.

The aims of this part of the examination are:
• to make the horse breathe deeply and rapidly and to increase the heart rate so that abnormalities of the heart and lungs can be detected
• to work the horse sufficiently hard so that any undetected injuries show up as lameness or stiffness after a period of rest.

A riding horse is usually observed at walk and trot on a 20 m circle. One or two 10 m circles are included on both reins. The horse is then asked to canter for 5–10 minutes, passing close to the vet on each circuit. Any unusual respiratory noises are noted.

The speed is then increased to a controlled gallop.

The heart rate and rhythm, and rate and depth of breathing are recorded immediately the horse is pulled up.

The horse is then untacked and returned to the stable.

Young, unbroken horses or tiny ponies may be lunged. Pregnant mares are excluded from this part of the examination.

4) *A period of rest*

During the next half hour, the horse is allowed to rest. The slowing of the heart and respiratory rate is monitored. Meanwhile, the horse's identification and other details are recorded.

5) *Second trot and foot examination*

The horse is walked and trotted up. It is then turned in a tight circle on both reins and walked backwards. Its feet are re-examined with hoof testers and the flexion tests may be repeated.

At the end of the examination, the vet will advise on the suitability, or otherwise, of the horse for your requirements. If the clinical findings give any cause for concern, x-rays or endoscopy may be necessary before the vet can give a final opinion.

X-rays

These are recommended if:
• the clinical examination makes the vet suspicious that there may be a problem
• the feet are of unequal size or poor conformation.

Some prospective purchasers request foot x-rays as part of the routine examination. In these cases it is important that the limitations of radiography are understood and accepted.

For instance, minor changes may be seen in the navicular bone, but not all of these horses will go on to develop navicular disease. It is not possible to predict whether there will be further changes leading to clinical signs.

Endoscopy

Endoscopy is recommended if the horse makes a noise at exercise or allergic respiratory disease is suspected.

Blood tests

These may be taken as a routine check on the horse's health or to test for the presence of anti-inflammatory drugs.

Blood Testing

Blood tests are taken:
- as part of a routine health check
- to provide more information where the cause of the horse's illness is obscure
- to confirm or eliminate a clinical diagnosis.

Taking blood samples

Blood is obtained from the jugular vein in the horse's neck (*Figure 19.2*).

Samples for routine haematology must be taken when the horse is relaxed and before

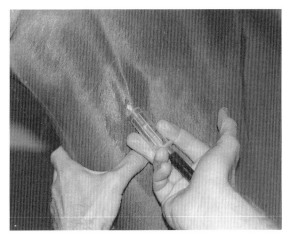

Figure 19.2 *Taking a blood sample*

exercise. This is because when the horse is excited, the spleen contracts and pushes a reserve pool of red blood cells into the circulation. The artificially high result could result in a mild anaemia being missed.

The components of blood

Blood is made up of:
- red blood cells – which transport oxygen to the tissues
- white blood cells – which defend the body against infection. There are five different types:
  - neutrophils
  - lymphocytes
  - eosinophils
  - monocytes
  - basophils
- platelets – which play an important role in the clotting mechanism of blood.

All these are suspended in a fluid known as plasma. Substances such as hormones, digested food and waste products are carried round the body in the plasma.

Haematology

Haematology is the study of blood. It includes the following measurements.

PCV – Packed Cell Volume

The percentage volume of whole blood that is taken up by red blood cells.

RBC – Red Blood Cell Count

The number of red blood cells $\times 10^{12}$ per litre of blood.

Hb – Haemoglobin

Haemoglobin is an iron-containing compound inside the red blood cells. It combines with oxygen in the air sacs of the lungs and transports it to the tissues. Carbon dioxide is transported in the opposite direction.

WBC – White Blood Cell Count

Total and differential white cell counts are recorded.

Interpretation of test results

There is no single normal value for these tests. Each laboratory has a normal range.

Red cell values

A low RBC, PCV, or Hb indicates the horse is anaemic. Higher than normal values are suggestive of excitement, dehydration or toxic shock.

The type of animal and its level of fitness are considered when the results are interpreted. For example, a PCV of 35 is acceptable for a child's pony at grass but it is low for a racehorse in training.

White cell values

The *total white cell count* is a useful indicator of the presence of infection. As a general rule the following apply.
- Bacterial infections usually result in a high total white cell count.
- In the early stages of a viral infection there is often a low white cell count. As the horse recovers the white cell count may rise above the normal range.

- Overwhelming infections, e.g. peritonitis, often result in a very low white cell count.

Deviation of a particular type of white cell from the normal range can also provide useful information.

Neutrophils (PMN – polymorphonuclear leucocytes)

These rise in number in response to bacterial infection. They are able to migrate from the small blood vessels into connective tissue where they kill and engulf bacteria. In severe, overwhelming infections, their numbers may be low.

Lymphocytes

These cells are important for recognising antigens such as viruses, bacteria and fungi. They stimulate antibody production. Lymphocytes may increase in number during the recovery phase of a viral infection.

Eosinophils

Eosinophils, monocytes and basophils are present in much smaller numbers.

Eosinophils increase with allergic and parasitic conditions.

Monocytes

The numbers increase in the presence of tissue damage or infection.

They migrate from the blood into the tissues and become transformed into large macrophages which engulf and digest bacteria, viruses and dead tissue.

Basophils

The numbers of basophils are too small for their significance to be fully understood. They are thought to be involved in allergic and inflammatory conditions.

Platelets

A platelet count is not included in a routine haematological examination.

Biochemistry

Biochemical tests are carried out on serum or plasma. They provide a great deal of information about what is happening in different parts of the horse's body. Variations from the normal range point to problems in specific organs so they can be a valuable aid to diagnosis. The following are a few examples, in alphabetical order.

Alkaline Phosphatase (SAP)

Levels of SAP are raised with:
- chronic liver disease
- intestinal problems
- abnormal bone metabolism.

As this test is not specific, the results are used in conjunction with the clinical findings and other test results to pinpoint the problem.

Aspartate Aminotransferase (AST, AAT, SGOT)

Levels are raised with:
- acute liver damage
- muscle damage.

Creatine Kinase (CK)

CK is raised when muscle damage occurs.

Creatinine

Raised where there is kidney damage.

Gamma Glutamyltransferase (GGT)

Gamma GT increases in cases of chronic liver damage.

Glutamate Dehydrogenase (GLDH)

Raised with acute liver damage.

Intestinal Phosphatase (IAP)

Raised with intestinal damage.

Proteins

Plasma proteins include:

Albumin

Low albumin can be indicative of malnutrition, liver, kidney or gut damage.

Globulin

The globulin can be separated into several fractions by a process called protein electrophoresis.

Increases in the different fractions indicate the following:

Alpha 2 – tissue damage

Beta 1 – damage from migrating *Strongylus vulgaris* larvae
Beta 2 – liver damage
Gamma globulins – bacterial or viral infection

IgG

This test is used to measure the level of immunity the foal receives from the maternal colostrum. It is usually performed when the foal is two days old.

Plasma Fibrinogen

Raised where tissue damage is present.

Urea

Raised when the kidneys are not functioning normally.

X-Rays

X-rays are taken when damage to bone is suspected, e.g. following lameness or injury. They show changes in the bone such as:
- fractures
- degenerative joint disease (arthritis)
- infection
- alteration in bone density.

They are often necessary for an accurate diagnosis to be made.

Radiation safety

Modern x-ray machines are fitted with a device called a light beam diaphragm. A beam of light shows exactly where the x-rays are going. This is an important safety feature and it also aids accurate positioning of the horse.

Lead aprons and gloves must be worn to protect the body from small amounts of scatter radiation.

Pregnant women and children must not assist with this procedure.

Procedure

X-rays may be taken with a mobile machine brought to your yard or at a veterinary hospital. In certain cases, a particularly powerful unit is required and the horse will have to visit a specialist centre.

The advantages of attending a veterinary hospital is that the x-ray films are developed immediately. If further views are required, they can be taken there and then.

Requirements for taking x-rays

If the x-ray machine is brought to your yard, the vet will require:
- A power point.
- A darkened stable so that the light beam can be seen.
- A smooth, flat surface, with plenty of room available for manoeuvring the x-ray machine around the patient.
- An experienced handler.
- A second assistant to position the limb and hold the x-ray plate.
- The part of the horse being radiographed *must* be clean and dry. Mud, kaolin and water show up on radiographs and may render the films useless.
- The horse may be sedated as any movement affects the quality of the radiographs. The equipment could easily be damaged by restless or nervous horses.
- Foot x-rays require special preparation. It is usually necessary for the shoes to be removed. The feet must be picked out and

scrubbed with a stiff brush to remove every trace of dirt.

These preparations should be made before the vet arrives.

Nerve Blocks

Injection of a small amount of local anaesthetic around a sensory nerve causes the area it supplies to become numb.

Nerve blocks are useful for:
- minor surgical procedures
- diagnosing some types of lameness.

Diagnosis of lameness

Where the cause of lameness is not obvious from the clinical examination, nerve blocks may help the vet to reach a diagnosis. The horse must be sufficiently lame that a difference in gait can be seen following the nerve block.

Procedure

The usual procedure is to start at the foot and work upwards. At each site the hair is clipped and the skin is sterilized before the injection is made.

Local anaesthetic can also be injected into joint spaces or around a lesion such as a splint that is suspected of causing lameness.

Restraint

The horse must be restrained with a bridle

and a twitch. This allows accurate positioning of the needle and reduces the risk of sudden movements which could cause the needle to break.

Time

Each nerve block takes 5–20 minutes to develop. The whole procedure may take a couple of hours.

The vet is unlikely to have time to do a full set of nerve blocks at the initial examination. Arrangements are usually made for a second visit or for the horse to go to the surgery.

Interpretation

If the horse becomes sound, the painful site has been desensitised. The cause of the lameness is within the last area of the limb to be blocked.

Where the lameness improves but is not completely eliminated, the vet will interpret the result using the clinical findings of the individual case.

Ultrasound Scanning

The ultrasound scanner provides the vet with valuable information when assessing ligament and tendon injuries. It can also be used to examine lungs and abdominal contents, e.g. a developing fetus.

Ultra-high frequency sound waves are used to produce an image on a screen. This is photographed and the prints are kept as a permanent record. They can be used to monitor the healing of an injury.

Image interpretation – tendons

Normal tendons look quite uniform in density, whereas a damaged tendon appears to have black holes within its substance.

Ultrasound scanning reveals the extent of an injury. The tendon is usually rescanned to check that healing is complete before the horse is returned to work.

General Anaesthesia

A horse may need to have a general anaesthetic for a routine operation planned in advance, or in an emergency (*Figure 19.3*).

Whenever possible, horses are anaesthetised at a premises with special operating facilities and a padded recovery box.

Preparing for an operation

Notification of the insurance company

The first action to take is notification of your insurance company.

It is advisable to discuss the details of any operation with the insurers before the surgery is undertaken. Some policies include general anaesthesia in the veterinary cover; others require payment of an additional premium at the time.

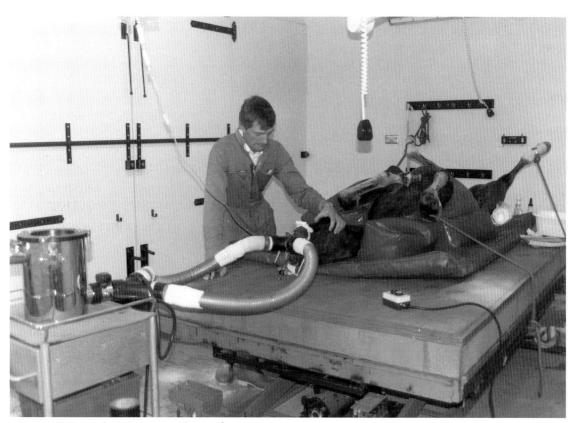

Figure 19.3   *A foal under general anaesthesia*

When an emergency arises out of office hours, the insurance company must be notified at the earliest opportunity after the event.

Starving the horse

With the exception of emergency situations, horses are starved for 12–18 hours before a general anaesthetic. This ensures the stomach is relatively empty and eliminates the small risk of a full stomach rupturing if the horse goes down awkwardly.

Removal of shoes

Shoes are routinely removed before a horse is anaesthetised. This is to prevent the horse damaging itself or the padding of the recovery box when coming round from the anaesthetic.

The anaesthetic procedure

All horses are given a thorough health check before being anaesthetised and blood tests may be taken. This is to make sure there are no other problems which require special attention or increase the likelihood of complications.

The horse is then given a sedative to make it quiet and relaxed.

When the sedative has taken effect, the anaesthetic is administered. The vet injects the drug(s) through a catheter placed in the jugular vein.

Once the horse is unconscious, anaesthesia is maintained by further infusion of drugs into the bloodstream, or by inhalation of anaesthetic gas through a tube placed in the trachea. This continues while the operation is in progress.

As soon as the operation is finished, the horse is allowed to come round. It is kept under observation until safely back on its feet.

Euthanasia

Having a horse put down is a problem that all owners may have to face. Euthanasia may be planned in advance or carried out as an emergency.

The most common reasons include:
- prevention of suffering, e.g. with an incurable and painful disease or following a serious injury
- ending the life of an old horse or pony
- economic considerations, e.g. when a horse is no longer capable of fulfilling the activities for which it was purchased.

Advance considerations

Notification of the insurance company

If the horse is the subject of an insurance claim, the company must be notified. With the exception of emergency situations, the permission of the insurers is needed to put the horse down.

Location

The full carcass value can only be obtained by taking the horse to an abattoir. It *must* be fit to travel and free from medication or any condition that makes the carcass unfit for human consumption.

Many owners have their horses put down at home. The horse is in familiar surroundings and does not experience any stress.

Disposal of the carcass

In many cases, the carcass goes to the local hunt kennels.

However, when the horse has been euthanased by injection of anaesthetic, the meat is unsuitable for feeding. In these cases the carcass must be buried in a suitable site approved by The National Rivers Authority.

Procedure

Using a gun

The vet or the local huntsman may euthanase the horse using a gun or captive bolt pistol. This is the quickest method. The horse dies instantly although reflex movements occur for a couple of minutes.

By injection

An alternative method is to give the horse an overdose of anaesthetic by intravenous injection. This method is less popular because of the problem of carcass disposal. However, there are some situations (e.g. crowded public places) when using a gun is undesirable.

20 Further Advice and Practical Tips

Horse Insurance

Insurance is a very competitive business. Most equine magazines have several advertisements, and each company claims to have the best policy.

There is no legal requirement to hold horse insurance, although it is advisable to have Public Liability cover. This insures against claims and legal costs arising from damage or injuries caused by your horse. It is automatically provided with membership of the BHS, BSJA and the Pony Club.

The decision on whether or not to insure the horse – and the type of cover needed – must be made after weighing the risks against the costs.

The options

The options for cover include the following.
- Death from accident or illness including transit, foaling and humane destruction by a vet.

   Humane destruction can be defined as euthanasia that is carried out in order to prevent or end incurable and excessive suffering. It may be carried out as an emergency, e.g. with irreparable fractures, terminal colics and situations where the behaviour of the horse endangers human life.

   Alternatively, humane destruction may be proposed after the horse has failed to respond to treatment. This category includes severely lame horses which would require painkillers for the rest of their lives, or horses suffering from a progressive and incurable disease such as cancer.

   Humane destruction *does not* include horses that are 'pasture sound' but no longer able to perform the work required of them.

   With the exception of emergency situations, permission to carry out euthanasia must be sought from the insurance company. They may wish to obtain a second opinion and are quite within their rights to do so.
- Loss by theft/straying, including recovery fees.
- Hire of a replacement animal following theft.
- Public liability.
- Vet's fees. Cover against vet's fees is recommended. The horse may require several visits for a single illness or injury and the charges soon mount up.
- Permanent loss of use.

   'Permanent loss of use' means that the horse is rendered *permanently incapable* of fulfilling the function for which it is kept. Such loss cannot be claimed until appropriate treatment has been given and the horse has been allowed sufficient time to recover.

In these cases you have the option of keeping the horse as a hack or companion and being paid a percentage of the insured value.

- Personal accident.
- Dental treatment.
- Saddlery and tack.
- Loss of entry fees.
- Stable insurance cover.

In general, the more comprehensive the cover selected, the higher the premium.

It is advisable to select the type of cover you require and obtain quotes from several companies. Before making a decision, read the small print and check the details.

Applying for insurance cover

The insurance company requires assurance that the horse is in good health at the inception of the policy. Conditions that are present at the time the policy is taken out may be excluded from the cover.

An owner's declaration of health is included on the proposal form. All the questions must be answered truthfully or the policy will be invalid.

Some companies require a veterinary surgeon's certificate of health. For horses over a certain value and policies including 'Permanent loss of use', a five-stage vetting certificate is usually required.

Points to consider when taking out a policy

Cost and type of cover

The cost varies with the value and proposed use of the horse. A riding horse is less likely to be injured than a three-day eventer and the premium is adjusted accordingly.

Be realistic about the level of cover you need and select a policy that gives you peace of mind at a price you can afford. Some spread the payment into instalments paid by direct debit or post-dated cheques.

Discounts

A number of companies offer a no-claims bonus and discounts for freeze-marked horses or the provision of recent vetting certificates and clean x-rays.

Date the cover commences

The cover may not commence until 14 days after the policy is taken out, leaving you uninsured for this period.

Exclusions and excess charges

Check the small print for specific exclusions such as surgical operations – some policies require payment of an additional premium should the occasion arise.

Most have an excess charge, so that you pay, for example, the first £50 of any claim.

Level of cover against vet's fees

Check the level of cover provided. In six policies selected at random, the vet's fees cover ranged from £150–£2,000 per incident. £2,000 will cover the cost of colic surgery, whereas £150 covers little more than the initial visit, drugs and diagnostic tests.

Limits on claims

Some companies impose an upper limit on total claims within the insurance period.

Reputation

It is worth asking the vet and other contacts in the equine world for their experience of the proposed insurance company – does it handle claims promptly and fairly?

Making a claim

As soon as the horse becomes ill or is injured, the insurance company must be notified. This applies even if you do not have cover for veterinary fees or if the injury is minor and unlikely to exceed the policy excess.

This ensures that in the event of an apparently simple case becoming more serious, the insurers can be certain the horse has received appropriate veterinary treatment from the start.

It may be useful to record details of the vet's visits, telephone conversations and letters sent, in a diary for future reference.

A claim form is sent for completion by the owner and the vet. The vet fills in details concerning the diagnosis, treatment and costs and sends it back to the insurance company.

A veterinary certificate may be required at the end of treatment stating that the horse has made a full recovery.

Second Opinions

In some circumstances you or the vet may decide that a second opinion would be of value. Obtaining and providing second opinions is part of a vet's everyday routine; it causes no annoyance or offence.

The horse may be referred to a veterinary school or hospital for more specialised tests, or to a colleague with wide experience in the particular field.

The vet will make all the arrangements and provide an up-to-date case history. This will include blood test results, x-rays and details of any medication.

The correct procedure

When obtaining a second opinion, the correct procedure must be followed. This is laid out in the Code of Professional Conduct for Veterinary Surgeons.

It states that once an animal has been examined by a vet, no other vet is allowed to examine or treat the animal without the prior consent of the vet in charge of the case.

Apart from professional courtesy, these rules are made for the welfare of the animal. In the absence of the case history, medication may be unnecessarily repeated or incompatible drugs given.

Box Rest

Box rest means confinement of the horse to a stable. This may be for a few days or several weeks, depending on the severity of the injury.

Objective

The purpose is to prevent uncontrolled exercise and allow an injury to heal. Stabling virtually eliminates the risk of further damage.

With a programme of care and rest, many horses with minor strains and sprains make a full recovery.

Management of the horse

Change of routine

Owners are often concerned that the horse will become distressed by the change in routine. However, even the most highly-strung horse soon settles down. If necessary, sedative tablets may be used for the first few days.

Feeding – concentrates

Very little concentrate feed is needed except in the case of pregnant mares.

Too much hard feed in the diet with little or no exercise can lead to serious conditions including laminitis and lymphangitis. Discuss the diet with your vet.

Feeding – hay

Good quality hay should form the bulk of the ration.

As many horses develop an allergic cough when confined to the stable, the hay should be soaked for several hours to reduce the number of inhaled fungal spores.

Ventilation

Special attention should be paid to the ventilation of the box, so the horse has plenty of fresh air.

Exercise

Turning out even the most sensible horse for a short period while on box rest may result in further injury and is never worth the risk.

In some cases the vet will recommend that the horse is walked out in hand for a specified length of time each day. Always use a bridle and lunge rein to minimise the chance of the horse getting away from you.

Bedding

The horse needs a comfortable bed. This should be kept scrupulously clean to minimise odours, mould growth and the risk of thrush infection. Horses that eat straw bedding should be kept on wood shavings or paper to reduce the risk of colic.

If a second stable is available, it can be used during the day. This allows both to be kept thoroughly clean.

Care of the feet

The feet must be picked out twice daily and carefully inspected for the first sign of thrush. Regular trimming by the farrier is just as important as when the horse is in work.

Boredom

Horses, like people, are individuals. Some are happier left undisturbed in a quiet corner, while others enjoy watching the activities of a busy yard.

Offering small quantities of hay throughout the day helps to relieve the boredom. If necessary, toys or a companion can be provided.

Understandably, many owners dislike the thought of the horse being confined for 24 hours a day. If you feel unable to cope with the situation, send the horse to a well-run livery yard for the period of enforced rest.

Turning out

Special care should be taken when turning the horse out for the first time after box rest. The following steps should be followed.
1) Use a suitable paddock with good fencing and plenty of grass. Avoid hilly, uneven or stony ground.
2) Choose a quiet time of day.
3) Do not give the horse a feed beforehand, so it will be inclined to graze rather than gallop.
4) If considered necessary, arrange for the vet to administer a sedative injection. Once the sedative has taken effect, lead the horse carefully and avoid making any sharp turns as it is likely to be a little uncoordinated.
5) With a bridle on top of a headcollar, lead the horse to the middle of the field and allow it to graze in hand for a few minutes. When the horse seems relaxed, gently slip the bridle off and move away immediately as it may buck and kick in excitement.
6) Leave the horse by itself or with a sensible companion. Check on it throughout the day.

Rehabilitation

Depending on the nature of the injury, a programme of controlled exercise is often necessary to bring the horse back to full work.

Freeze Marking

Freeze marking is a method of giving your horse a clear and permanent identification number. The characters are marked on the left side of the saddle region or left shoulder using a very cold instrument. The pigment cells are killed and the new hair growth is white (*Figure 20.1*).

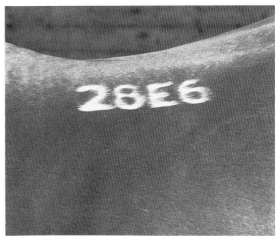

Figure 20.1   *A freeze mark*

Grey horses are identified using the same technique but a bald mark is created, usually on the shoulder.

A registration and identification certificate is sent to you before the operator's visit. The horse's details must be filled in so the operator can check them before allocating a number.

The initial fee covers the horse while it remains in your ownership. There is no annual charge.

Branding procedure

Freeze marking is not painful but it does give an unpleasant sensation while the chilled markers are held in place. The horse should therefore be restrained in a stable or holding pen by an experienced adult.

Over the next few weeks the dead hair and skin fall away. The mark becomes bald and looks very pink. In time this will be covered with white hair. The freeze mark takes 3–4 months to develop.

Aftercare

A 4–7 day rest is recommended, though some horses remain sensitive for up to three weeks. It is therefore sensible to arrange the procedure for a time when an enforced rest would not disrupt your plans. The horse may be lunged during the recovery period.

Try to use rugs which do not require a roller immediately after freeze marking. If a roller is used, place plenty of padding underneath.

Always use a clean, thick numnah while the freeze mark is forming.

A long coat may obscure bald marks during the winter months. This is easily remedied by clipping the area.

Advantages

- Horse thieves are less likely to steal a freeze-marked animal.
- If the horse is stolen it can be easily and positively identified.
- The freeze-mark company liaise with the police and coordinate the search for a stolen horse. Ports, slaughterhouses and horse sales are notified. A 24 hour service is provided.
- A substantial reward is offered for information leading to conviction of a person stealing a freeze-marked horse.
- Some insurance companies offer a reduction in premium if the horse is freeze-marked.

Restraint of the Horse

Most horses tolerate a wide variety of treatments when held in a headcollar by a quiet, competent handler.

However, in situations where the horse is frightened or in pain, additional restraint may be necessary to ensure:

- efficient, accurate treatment
- the safety of everyone present.

The following methods can be used:

- confinement to a restricted space
- bridling
- holding a leg up
- using a twitch
- sedation
- general anaesthesia.

Use of a stable or holding pen

Many horses move away from a person cleaning a wound or administering a treatment. When confined in a loosebox, the animal will usually move against the wall and then stand quietly and accept the procedure.

Using a stable eliminates interference from other horses and ponies.

Use of a bridle

Strong, excitable or aggressive horses should wear a bridle to maximise control and safety.

Holding a leg up

Lifting a forelimb makes it more difficult for the horse to move or kick out.

When you are attending to a hind limb injury, the forelimb on the same side should be lifted by an assistant.

If you are both on one side of the horse, the handler can pull its head towards you if it lashes out. The quarters will then swing in the opposite direction.

When dealing with a forelimb injury, the opposite forelimb should be lifted.

Using a twitch

The twitch (*Figure 20.2*) is used when the aforementioned methods of restraint have proved inadequate. In most cases it enables

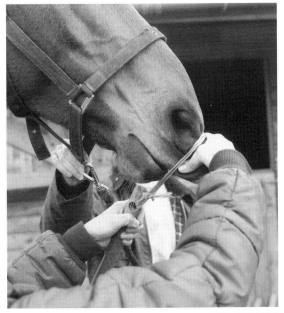

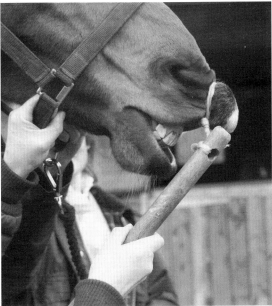

Figure 20.2 *Applying a twitch. The loop is placed over the horse's upper lip* (above), *then twisted until secure* (below)

treatment to proceed without further problems.

A twitch can be made from a piece of cotton rope or a double thickness of baler twine attached to part of an old broom handle. The loop of twine is placed over the horse's upper lip and twisted until secure. Metal twitches can be purchased from most saddlers.

Application of the twitch usually causes the horse to go into a sleepy, trance-like state. The head droops and the eyes may close. The horse becomes less sensitive to painful stimuli. This is due to the release from the brain of very powerful painkillers called endorphins.

A similar effect is achieved by twisting an ear or grasping and twisting a fold of skin from the neck. The latter technique is particularly useful when handling foals and yearlings.

When using a twitch, keep the stable door closed but not bolted. It is very important for handlers to be able to leave the box quickly when dealing with a fractious horse.

Important note: a few horses become more violent when a twitch is used. If the horse rears or strikes out, do not proceed. Remove the twitch at once.

Sedation

Where physical methods of restraint have failed, arrange for the vet to administer a sedative.

A number of sedative drugs are available. They may be used singly or in various combinations, depending on the degree of sedation required. Some also have analgesic properties.

The degree of sedation depends on:
- the drug(s) used
- the dose
- the temperament of the horse
- the horse's level of excitement at the time the drug is administered; sedatives work most effectively when given to a calm, relaxed horse.

They are usually given by intramuscular or intravenous injection. ACP (acepromazine) is also available in tablet and paste forms for oral administration.

Examples of situations requiring sedation include:
- treatment of painful wounds
- teeth rasping and clipping of head-shy horses
- minor surgical procedures, e.g. wart removal
- turning a horse out after a prolonged period of box rest.

General anaesthesia

When it is essential for the horse to remain completely still, the horse is given a general anaesthetic.

Taking a Horse's Temperature

The normal temperature of the horse is 38 °C (100.5 °F). However, many healthy horses have a temperature as low as 37 °C (98.5 °F). Temperatures up to 38.5 °C (101.5 °F) are acceptable on hot days or after exercise.

Procedure

Unless the horse is familiar with the procedure, it should be held by an assistant.
1) Shake the thermometer until the mercury is below the temperature scale.
2) Lubricate the bulb with Vaseline or saliva.
3) Run your hand over the horse's quarters and lift the tail.
4) Stand close to the horse and to one side. Gently slide the bulb through the anal opening until two thirds of the thermometer is inside the rectum.
5) Tilt the thermometer so the bulb lies in contact with the rectal wall.
6) Wait a full minute.
7) Withdraw the thermometer and wipe it clean.
8) Read the temperature.
9) Shake the thermometer until the mercury is below the start of the temperature scale.
10) Clean the thermometer with disinfectant and cold water before returning it to its case.
11) Store the thermometer in a cool place.

How to Take a Horse's Pulse

The resting pulse rate of a horse is 30–40 beats per minute. The pulse rate increases:
- with exercise or excitement
- when the horse has a temperature
- with acute pain.

Procedure

The easiest place to take a pulse is where the facial artery passes under the lower jaw (*Figure 20.3*). The horse must not be chewing as this makes it very difficult to locate.
1) Run your fingers along the lower edge of the mandible. The artery can be felt as a tubular structure.
2) Apply *light* pressure with the flat of your first three fingers.
3) Feel the pulse.
4) Count the number of beats in a fifteen-second period.

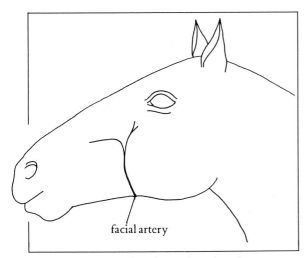

facial artery

Figure 20.3   *Site for taking a horse's pulse*

5) Multiply this number by four to obtain the horse's pulse rate.

Intramuscular Injections

Whenever possible, injections are administered by the vet. However, when the horse needs a course of treatment, the owner or an experienced person at the yard may give intramuscular injections.

Intravenous injections must always be given by the vet.

When injecting a horse, sterility is essential. If the contents of the bottle, the syringe or the needle become contaminated, discard them immediately.

Preparing the horse

The horse should be:
- clean and dry; never inject a horse through a wet, muddy coat

- adequately restrained: tying the horse up is not recommended. It is much more likely to move or pull back than if held by an assistant.

Loading the syringe

1) Wash your hands.
2) Check the contents of the bottle and read the instructions.
3) Shake the bottle thoroughly.
4) Wipe the rubber stopper of the bottle with a piece of cotton wool soaked in surgical or methylated spirit.
5) Place a sterile needle, still in its cover, onto a sterile syringe. Remove the needle cover. *If the needle is dropped or accidentally touches anything, discard it and use another one.*
6) Hold the bottle upside down and push the needle through the rubber stopper. Check that the point of the needle is below the fluid level and withdraw the plunger (*Figure 20.4*).
7) Withdraw a little more treatment than is

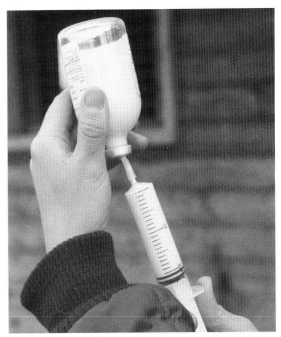

Figure 20.4   *Filling the syringe*

required. With the syringe still in the upright position, return the excess to the bottle. This removes any air bubbles.
8) Replace the needle cover.
9) If any of the drug spills on your hands, wash it off immediately.

Common difficulties

A considerable volume of air enters the syringe when the plunger is withdrawn

There are two likely explanations.
- The top of the needle is intermittently protruding above the fluid level in the bottle.
- Air is being drawn in at the join between the needle and syringe. Tightening the connection eliminates the problem.

Withdrawing the drug is difficult and requires a very strong pull on the plunger.

This is especially common with thick antibiotic suspensions. There are two tips.
- In cold weather, warm the antibiotic to blood heat (no hotter). Either stand the bottle in a bowl of lukewarm water for a few minutes or keep the drug indoors.
- Inject a volume of air into the bottle that is equivalent to the amount of treatment required before withdrawing the drug.

Injection Technique

Selecting the site

There are several suitable muscle sites but the muscle of the neck is advised for the less experienced. The site for injection is a hand's breadth up from the base of the neck, halfway between the crest and the underside of the neck (*Figure 20.5*).

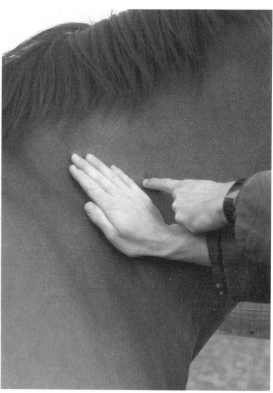

Figure 20.5   *The recommended site for intramuscular injections*

Young foals are not injected in the neck as any subsequent stiffness will discourage them from sucking. The rump or the back of the thigh are the sites that are most commonly used. Expert restraint is absolutely essential.

The chosen site may be swabbed with surgical or methylated spirit.

Giving the injection

Method 1

1) Remove the needle from the loaded syringe and hold it between the thumb and first two fingers. Remove the cap.
2) Tap the horse with the back of the hand close to the injection site (*Figure 20.6*). Insert the needle smartly in a horizontal direction to its full depth.

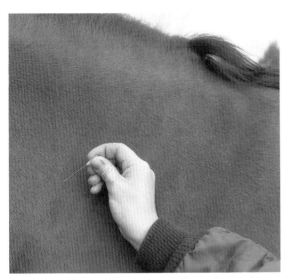

Figure 20.6 *Tap the horse with the back of your hand before inserting the needle*

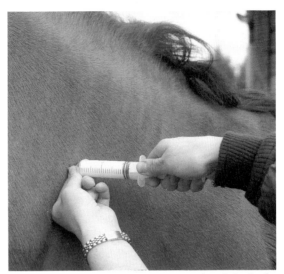

Figure 20.8 *Attach the syringe and pull back the plunger to check that no blood enters the syringe*

3) *Check that no blood fills or drips from the hub of the needle (Figure 20.7). If it does, the tip of the needle has entered a blood vessel and must be repositioned before the injection is given.*

4) Attach the loaded syringe. Pull the plunger back to check that no blood is drawn into the syringe before proceeding any further (*Figure 20.8*).

5) Depress the plunger to give the injection. Considerable pressure may be required to inject thick antibiotic suspensions. In order to avoid the needle and syringe being forced apart, hold their joint with the thumb and forefinger of the left hand (*Figure 20.9*).

6) Withdraw the needle. Do not be alarmed if there is a trickle of blood from the injection site.

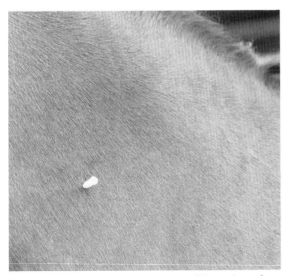

Figure 20.7 *Check that no blood fills or drips from the hub of the needle before attaching the syringe*

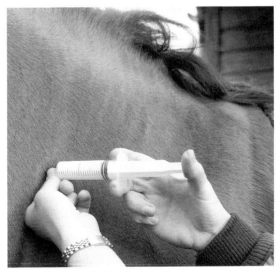

Figure 20.9 *Giving the injection*

7) Do not pat the horse on the injection site as it is likely to be tender.
8) Use alternate sides of the neck for each injection if several days treatment is prescribed.
9) Always complete the course of injections, even if the horse appears to have recovered.

Method 2

This technique is especially useful for young and fractious animals.
1) Leave the needle attached to the loaded syringe and remove the cap.
2) With the left hand, grasp a fold of skin close to the injection site (*Figure 20.10*).
3) Gently, but deliberately, guide the needle through the skin, deep into the muscle.
4) Pull the plunger back to check the needle has not entered a blood vessel then proceed with the injection.

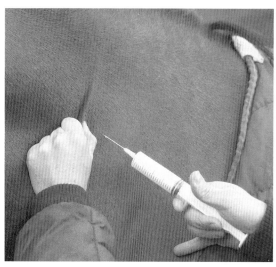

Figure 20.10   *Alternative method of giving an injection*

Possible complications

- *The needle drops into the bed and cannot be found.* The relevant area of bedding must be removed and searched.

- *The horse is uncooperative.* Use further restraint, e.g. a twitch. If the horse is still difficult and you feel you are unlikely to be successful, do not continue. Allow the horse to relax and seek experienced help.
- *Blood appears in the hub of the needle or the syringe* when the plunger is withdrawn. **Do not inject the treatment.** Some substances such as antibiotic suspensions are lethal if accidentally injected into a blood vessel. Remove the needle and start again.
- *If the needle breaks*, grasp and withdraw the protruding part of the needle. If this is not possible, mark the spot and seek professional help.
- *The horse may develop a stiff neck* which prevents lowering of the head to graze or drink. Feed and water must be raised. Hot fomentations help to ease the stiffness. Inform the vet, who may prescribe phenylbutazone to reduce the inflammation and discomfort.
- *An abscess may develop at the injection site.* This may be due to non-sterile technique, but can also occur in spite of careful preparation. Contact the vet.

Disposal of needles and syringes

Never throw used needles and syringes into the dustbin. Return them to the vet's surgery.

Partially used bottles of treatment can be stored for a short period of time, provided the contents are sterile. Do not use them to treat another horse without prior consultation with the vet.

Storage of Medicines

Where medicines are kept in the first-aid kit

or are left over from a course of treatment, they should be stored correctly and safely.

Guidelines for storing medicines

- Medicines and dressings must be stored where they remain clean and are not contaminated by dust – a sealed tin or box within a cupboard is ideal.
- They should not be subjected to extremes of temperature. The storage area should be cool, dark and dry. *Always keep them out of direct sunlight and away from radiators.* Very few medicines require storage in the fridge.
- Keep them out of reach of children and animals. Drugs should, ideally, be stored in a locked cupboard.
- Each medicine must be labelled with:
  - the name and address of the veterinary practice
  - the date the drug was supplied
  - the name of the drug
  - the correct dose
  - the method of administration
  - the duration of treatment
  - the name of the horse for which the treatment is prescribed.

Disposal of medicines

Some drugs cannot be stored once the container has been opened. Unfinished bottles and tubes must be disposed of safely. Contact your vet for advice.

Discard out-of-date drugs and dressings. The expiry date is usually printed on the container.

Hygiene

Take care not to contaminate tubs of ointment that are used over a period of time. Wash your hands thoroughly each time ointment is removed.

Veterinary Records

A written record should be kept of all treatment, including routine worming and vaccinations, that each horse receives.

These records should be stored in the tack room or office where they are readily to hand.

It is advisable for owners of livery yards to have *written permission* to call the vet out to any horse left in their care. This ensures prompt veterinary attention if an emergency occurs and the owner cannot be contacted.

Drugs and the Competition Horse

The FEI has drawn up a list of Prohibited Substances. This is to ensure that horses compete on their individual merits and their performance is not improved by the use of drugs.

The rules prevent a horse which is receiving medication from being exposed to the stress of competition. They are made to protect the animal's wellbeing as well as ensuring that the competition is fair.

Prohibited substances

The list of prohibited substances includes

those acting on:
- the nervous system
- the cardiovascular system
- the respiratory system
- the alimentary system
- the urinary system
- the musculoskeletal system
- the immune system.

The list also includes the following groups of drugs:
- antibiotics, antibacterial and antiviral substances
- antiparasitic substances, i.e. wormers
- antipyretics, analgesics and anti-inflammatory substances other than phenylbutazone and oxyphenbutazone (a metabolite of phenylbutazone)
- endocrine secretions and their synthetic counterparts
- substances affecting blood coagulation
- cytotoxic substances.

Maximum permissible levels

There is an additional list of substances for which maximum permissible levels have been established.

Phenylbutazone: concentration of 2.0 micrograms per millilitre of plasma
Oxyphenbutazone: concentration of 2.0 micrograms per millilitre of plasma
Theobromine: concentration of 2.0 micrograms per millilitre of urine.
Salicylic acid: concentration of 750.0 micrograms per millilitre of urine.
Arsenic: concentration of 0.2 micrograms per millilitre of urine.

These FEI rules are enforced by most equestrian sporting bodies. One exception is the permitted use of phenylbutazone by the British Show Jumping Association.

Clearance time for drugs

The majority of drugs are eliminated from the horse's system within eight days. However, there is no guarantee that a drug will not be detectable after this period.

The clearance time is affected by factors such as dose, route of administration, diet, concurrent administration of other drugs and the individual horse's metabolism.

Medication of any sort should therefore be avoided when a competition date approaches. If treatment is unavoidable, consult your vet about the withdrawal time of the drugs and the advisability of competing.

Control of Fly Irritation

During the summer, flies cause a great deal of irritation to grazing animals.

The irritation can cause an animal to rub or nibble itself until sore. This may lead to loss of condition as well as skin lesions and the spread of disease.

The problems caused by flies

Flies bother the horse in various ways.

House flies gather in large numbers and feed on discharges from the eyes, nostrils and sheath. They introduce infection into wounds.

Stable flies breed in soiled bedding and their painful bite leaves a raised lump with a small scab.

Culicoides midges, active at dawn and dusk, cause sweet itch in susceptible animals.

Horse flies have a very painful bite. Some horses become anxious and gallop round the field trying to escape from them.

Bot flies irritate the horse as they lay their eggs.

Control of flies

Total fly control is virtually impossible, although some success is achieved with the following measures.

Fly deterrents

Fly repellent

This can be applied at regular intervals. Many different types are available from vets, saddlers and agricultural merchants. The instructions should be followed carefully.

It is advisable to test the product on a small area of skin (e.g. the inside of the horse's thigh) the day before treating the horse.

Insecticidal cream

Applied as a thin layer inside the ears, insecticidal cream discourages small black flies from feeding. Deposits of cream should not be allowed to build up or enter the ear canal. It can also be used on small wounds.

Insecticidal wound powder

This protects small cuts and grazes.

Insecticidal bands or cattle ear tags

These can be attached to the bridle or head-collar. The insecticide spreads over the skin surface.

Protective coverings

A fly fringe

A fly fringe attached to the headcollar prevents flies from feeding around the eyes and provides considerable relief (*Figure 20.11*).

Protective face and ear covers

These give excellent protection for short periods of time. However, flies can become trapped inside the material so the horse must be inspected regularly. They are easily torn and expensive to replace (*Figure 20.12*).

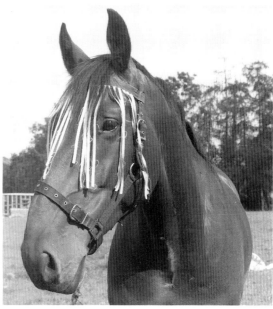

Figure 20.11   *Fly fringe: note the frayed edges on this fly fringe need trimming as they can also irritate the horse's eyes*

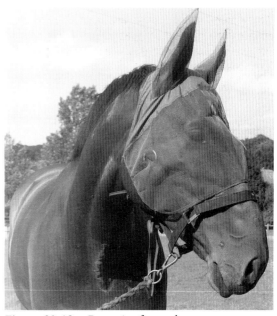

Figure 20.12   *Protective face and ear cover*

A summer sheet

This protects a large area of the horse from biting flies both in the field and when stabled.

Shelter

A cool, clean shelter

This is the most satisfactory method of fly control. During hot weather, horses benefit from being stabled by day and turned out at night.

The shelter should be sited as far as possible from fly breeding grounds such as stagnant water and the muck heap. Where there is no shelter available, the horse should have access to some shade.

Turning horses out in pairs is helpful as they can stand head to tail and flick the flies from each other.

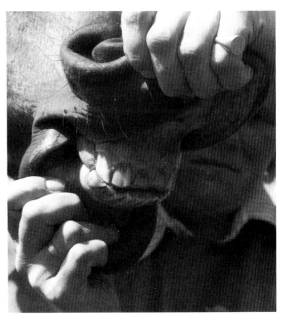

Figure 20.13 *Abnormally worn teeth in a crib biter*

Stable Vices

Stable vices are bad habits developed by horses and ponies, usually as a result of boredom. Once acquired they can be difficult to cure and may reduce significantly the horse's value. Since the behaviour is quickly copied by others, these animals are often unwelcome in livery yards.

Horses should not be confined to the stable for long periods of time without work. Where this is unavoidable due to injury, a companion such as a goat, sheep or Shetland pony may be provided. Some horses will play for hours with toys such as a large ball suspended from the roof inside a haynet.

Crib biting

Crib biters (*Figure 20.13*) chew fences, gates, and various parts of the stable. Over a period of time their incisor teeth wear abnormally. In severe cases the teeth no longer meet, making grazing difficult and thus leading to loss of condition.

Control

- If the habit only occurs in the stable, the horse should be turned out for as long as possible. Plenty of hay should be provided when the horse is brought in.
- Some horses only crib bite when being groomed or tacked up. This is easily overcome by tying the horse to a ring in a solid wall away from fences and other projections.
- The stable and fences should be regularly coated with creosote. 'Favourite' chewing spots can be liberally covered with unpleasant tasting preparations which are available from tack shops. A metal strip should be placed over the top of the stable door.

- Provision of toys or a companion may stop the behaviour.
- Ensure the horse's diet is balanced, and supply a mineral and salt lick.
- Fence chewing can be controlled by placing an electric fence inside the wooden one. Alternatively, an electrified wire can be run along the top of the fence.

Windsucking

The horse arches its neck, grasps a solid object (e.g. manger, fence, top of the stable door) then sucks in and swallows air with a gulping noise. Some horses windsuck without holding onto a fixed object.

Control

- The habit is controlled in many horses by fitting a wide leather strap around the top of the neck. Special collars are available with a metal piece under the throat. As the horse tries to arch its neck this digs into the muscle and causes discomfort. It does not interfere with eating or respiration (*Figure 20.14*).
- Forssell's operation involves removing a part of the sternothyrohyoideus and omohyoideus muscles on the underside of the horse's neck. The nerve supply is also cut. While the operation is a complete success with some horses, it does not improve others. The loss of muscle alters the outline of the horse's neck.

Weaving

The horse swings its head and neck from side to side while shifting its weight from one forelimb to the other. The front feet may be alternately lifted quite high off the ground.

Weaving usually takes place when the horse is looking out over the stable door, but some horses do it inside the stable or even when tied outside. The behaviour is associated with boredom or anxiety; it can cause loss of condition and muscle fatigue. The front shoes tend to wear very quickly.

Control

- The best solution to weaving is to turn the horse out.
- The habit may be controlled by fitting a V-shaped grille on the stable door (*Figure 20.15*). However, confirmed weavers often toss their heads up and down through the grille instead.
- The habit is copied quickly by other horses, so weavers should be stabled where they cannot be seen by their stable companions.

Box walking

Some horses compulsively walk round their boxes for many hours of the day. This behaviour can lead to loss of condition and makes it almost impossible to keep the bedding clean and fresh.

Control

Once the habit is established, it is very difficult to control. Provision of toys or a stable companion may help, but turning the horse out with a companion is often the only solution.

Rug tearing

When a horse starts to rip rugs with its teeth,

Figure 20.14
*Windsucking
collar*

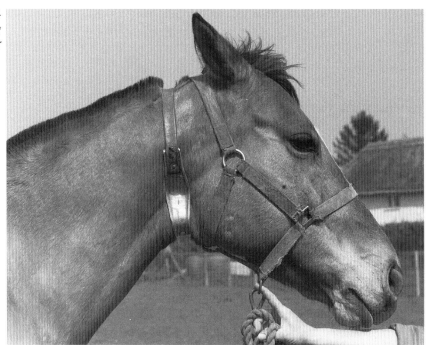

Figure 20.15
*A V-shaped grille may
stop a horse weaving*

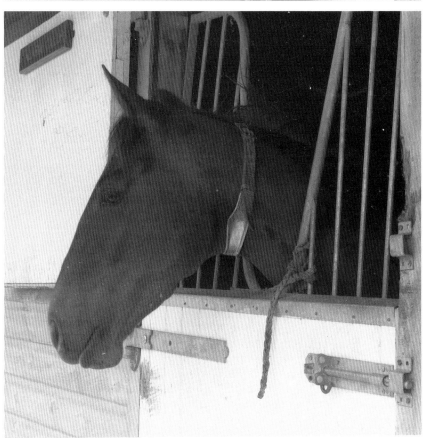

it may be due to boredom or discomfort.

Control

- Make sure the horse is not too hot.

- Check that the horse's roller is not uncomfortable or too tight. A rug with crossover surcingles may be preferred.
- Inspect the horse's coat for parasites such as lice.
- Provide something else for the horse to play with.

Further Reading

Horse Anatomy (1983), Peter C. Goody. London: J. A. Allen

Equine Nutrition and Feeding (1986), David Frape. Harlow: Longmans

Equine Injury and Therapy (1987), Mary Bromiley. Oxford: Blackwell Scientific

Hickman's Farriery (1988), John Hickman and Martin Humphreys. London: J. A. Allen

Veterinary Notes for Horse Owners (1989), Horace Hayes. London: Stanley Paul

The Horse from Conception to Maturity (1989, new edition 1992), P. D. Rossdale. London: J. A. Allen

Index